Living with P.C.O.S.

Polycystic Ovary Syndrome

Angela Boss • Evelina Weidman Sterling
with Richard S. Legro, M.D.

Addicus Books
Omaha, Nebraska

An Addicus Nonfiction Book

ISBN 1-886039-49-6
Cover design by Peri Paloni
Illustrations by Jack Kusler

This book is not intended to be a substitute for a physician, nor do the authors intend to give advice contrary to that of an attending physician.

Library of Congress Cataloging-in-Publication Data
Best-Boss, Angela.
   Living with P.C.O.S. : polycystic ovary syndrome / Angela Best-Boss,
Evelina Weidman Sterling, Richard S. Legro.
       p. cm.
"An Addicus nonfiction book."
Includes bibliographical references and index.
   ISBN 1-886039-49-6 (alk. paper)
   1. Stein-Leventhal syndrome. 2. Stein-Leventhal syndrome—Treatment.
I. Sterling, Evelina Weidman, 1970- II. Legro, Richard S., 1957- III.
Title.
   RG480.S7 B47 2000
   618.1'1—dc21   00-010670

Addicus Books, Inc.
P.O. Box 45327
Omaha, Nebraska 68145
Web site: http://www.AddicusBooks.com
Printed in the United States of America
10 9 8 7 6 5 4 3

To the glory of God for His gift
of Kaylyn and Clara

A.J.B.

To Dan, Benjamin, and Elena for
their love and support

E.W.S.

Contents

Foreword

PCOS women of the world unite! Finally, here is a readable and comprehensive book about polycystic ovary syndrome (PCOS) for women who suffer from its manifestations. This disorder has a tremendous impact on your image as a woman, your ability to reproduce, and ultimately on your long-term health. As such, PCOS is one of the most important issues in women's health.

This book has been a long time coming and is the first book about, by, and for PCOS women. It sheds the layers of complexity and medical doublespeak that shroud the syndrome. Unfortunately, this condition is both underdiagnosed and undertreated by many physicians. Part of the difficulty has been finding a universally accepted definition of the syndrome. Another part has been our ignorance as physicians about its fundamental cause. You, the women with PCOS, hold the key to unlocking these doors.

The greater attention that has been focused on PCOS in recent years is largely due to the advocacy of the women who suffer from the syndrome. It is due to their courage to come forward, and their hard work, that ever more public recognition and health research funding have been devoted to PCOS.

We, as physicians, can no longer ignore PCOS. We can no longer tell you to just shave. We can no longer tell you to just lose some weight. We can no longer tell you to just keep trying to get pregnant. We can no longer say don't worry about diabetes or heart disease or cancer. We must face PCOS, understand it, and treat it.

We, as researchers, cannot advance our understanding of PCOS without your advocacy and without your participation in our studies. For all your past, present, and future efforts in our studies and the studies of all who labor in this field: our collective thanks. I have received many awards and honors in my career, but the one of which I am proudest came from the Polycystic Ovarian Syndrome Association, Inc., for outstanding service to the support group. The award came from the heart from the women with PCOS. Again, my thanks and gratitude. We have only just begun.

Richard S. Legro, M.D.
Pennsylvania State University College of Medicine
Department of Obstetrics and Gynecology
M.S. Hershey Medical Center
Hershey, Pennsylvania

Preface

For most women with PCOS, there comes a time when you say, "Ah-ha! So *that's* what I have!" That epiphany began for me in 1998 on the night I happened to watch a network television program about PCOS. I was diagnosed officially several months later. I have what is a typical case, having displayed many of the symptoms since puberty. I gained weight early on and have always struggled with it. As a young woman, I had pleasant older physicians who said that some women just didn't have periods and that I would probably have difficulty getting pregnant.

Surprisingly, getting pregnant with my daughter Kaylyn couldn't have been easier. Having a second child has proved to be much more difficult. A few rounds of fertility medicines resulted in a second pregnancy, but an early miscarriage. Most recently, adding an insulin sensitizer has renewed my ovulatory cycles as well as my hope for another child.

This book is written out of a deep compassion for women with PCOS, their friends and family, and the medical professionals who treat them. For years, trying to find accurate information about PCOS has been difficult at best. We, the coauthors, have both been diagnosed with PCOS and wanted the best, most up-to-date information available about the disease and its treatment so that we could make informed medical choices.

Throughout the book, a number of wonderfully strong and courageous women share their stories. We are grateful for their gift. Their wisdom, insight, and experiences are equally as important as the medical community's offerings. These women are powerful reminders that as lonely as this journey can sometimes feel, many have walked before us.

Although living with PCOS is not necessarily easy, we now have access to a wider range of treatments than ever before. Additionally, with the growth of support chapters and Internet-based news groups and bulletin boards, there are thousands of women willing to walk with you. You are not alone.

A. Best-Boss

Ever since I was a teenager, I had always thought I had some kind of hormonal problem. When I told my doctor about my concerns, he told me to relax and my body would straighten itself out eventually. After that, I really didn't think about it too much until I wanted to have a baby.

My body never did straighten itself out. My symptoms only got worse. Since I had suspected all along that my hormones were not functioning properly, I made an appointment with an endocrinologist. Fortunately, he was very knowledgeable and immediately diagnosed me with PCOS. With the help of a fertility drug, Clomid, I was able to become pregnant twice and give birth to two beautiful children. I am just now coming to terms with my PCOS and how it affects my life. I continue to work with my doctors on an effective treatment plan that will hopefully help me live a long and healthy life.

E. Weidman Sterling

Introduction

My story may be something like yours. At age 13, I was slender and clear skinned. Then my body began to change. By 15, I had developed severe acne. By 17, I had suffered my first bout of depression. At 19, I began to notice excess body hair. At 21, I had an unusually large ovarian cyst that burst, putting me in the hospital. By 23, I had gone two years without a period and was beginning to have serious trouble maintaining my weight despite regular exercise and a low-fat diet.

Each step of the way, I consulted with medical professionals. In some cases I was given a nominal explanation and medication. In others, my concerns were abruptly dismissed. I was given birth control pills to control my irregular periods and told that I would need a "special pill" called Clomid to get pregnant. At 29 I tried to conceive and, happily, got pregnant on my fifth round of Clomid. I knew I had "women's problems" but, with that victory, figured I had them beat. Nowhere along the line was I ever told that I had polycystic ovary syndrome, let alone that I had a lifelong problem with vast implications for my health.

My first pregnancy was riddled with complications. Afterwards, I couldn't lose weight. I discovered that my triglycerides were soaring. Getting desperate, I tried fad diets such as the cabbage soup diet. When those didn't work, I experimented with vegetarianism and, strangely, actually gained weight! I read books on diet and exercise, diligently taking the advice in each book. Nothing worked.

Wanting a second child, I went to my gynecologist for more Clomid. Surprisingly, that didn't work either. No matter what I did, my body seemed to rebel.

Then one day, depressed and desperate, I searched the Internet and found the Polycystic Ovarian Syndrome Association (PCOSA). It was a revelation! My problems had a name! I began soaking up information. I learned about the insulin connection and that women with PCOS are at increased risk for diabetes and heart disease. Suddenly, what I had come to accept as just an aggravating female problem was much more.

I'll be honest, living with PCOS can be tough. But like so many challenges in life, it too has its rewards. I became active in the PCOSA, meeting others with PCOS and learning what I needed to take control of my health. Through education and sharing, I improved my physical and mental well-being and was finally able to conceive my desperately sought second child.

That is what this book is all about. It is a tool for you to gain the information you need to take control of PCOS. As you learn, rejoice in the knowledge that each day moves us closer to a treatment and, possibly, a cure. We are no longer in the dark! Just think, you and I could be the last generation of women affected by PCOS. A powerful thought indeed.

Kristin Hellman Rencher, Executive Director
Polycystic Ovarian Syndrome Association, Inc.

1

PCOS—A Complicated Disorder

As soon as Debbie hit puberty, her periods became irregular, she gained weight faster and easier than any of her girlfriends, and she was embarrassed by the amount of hair on her chin, arms, and legs. Her mother finally took her to the doctor, who brushed off the symptoms, explaining that it would take a while for her hormones to "adjust."

Debbie is now 28, happily married and ready to start a family. Unfortunately, she is still having the same problems. It seems her hormones still haven't "adjusted." As a matter of fact, it has been six months since her last period. When she talked to her doctor about this during her last visit, he indicated she may be under too much stress and that she is a few pounds overweight. The doctor said tests weren't necessary; it was nothing serious. Debbie should just go home and relax.

However, Debbie cannot relax. She is frustrated and confused. She knows *something* is wrong, but what?

What Is PCOS?

Polycystic ovary syndrome, or *PCOS*, is a complex hormone disorder that causes such symptoms as irregular menstrual cycles, infertility, excessive body hair, acne, and obesity. The syndrome is named for the tiny cysts that may form in the ovaries when the hormone imbalance interrupts the ovulation process. The term *polycystic* means "composed of many cysts." If the hormone imbalance is left untreated, the syndrome may lead to life-threatening illnesses such as diabetes, heart disease, stroke, and uterine and endometrial cancers.

Symptoms of PCOS

Because it is a syndrome, PCOS includes a set of symptoms. Women with PCOS can suffer from any combination of the symptoms listed here. Some women experience only one of these symptoms, while other women experience all of them. The severity of PCOS symptoms can vary widely from woman to woman. Talk to your physician if you suffer from one or more of these symptoms:

- Chronically irregular menstrual cycles or absent periods
- Infertility or difficulty conceiving (due to not ovulating)
- Obesity (greater than 20 percent over "ideal" weight)
- Sudden, unexplained weight gain (even if you are still of "normal" weight)
- Adult acne
- Excessive hair growth (especially dark hair on the face, chest, or abdomen)
- Male-pattern hair loss or thinning hair
- Type II diabetes or insulin resistance

It is possible to have the above symptoms and not have PCOS. However, most women with these symptoms, especially irregular menstrual cycles, do have PCOS. In fact, 80 percent of women with six or fewer periods per year have PCOS.

Researchers have found some variations in the symptoms among different races. For example, while excessive body hair is found among 70 percent of American women with PCOS, it only occurs in about 10 to 20 percent of Asian women. Unfortunately, there is not enough evidence to explain why these variations in symptoms occur.

Because the symptoms of PCOS can vary widely, it can be difficult to exclude or include symptoms as a part of the diagnosis. In fact, the World Health Organization tried to determine a comprehensive list of symptoms and couldn't agree on more than four of them. Further research is being done at a dozen facilities in the United States alone. There may be more common symptoms discovered as new studies are completed and women continue reporting their experiences.

Who Is Affected?

The most common endocrine disorder, PCOS is estimated to affect anywhere from 5 to 10 percent of all women. That means at least 5 million and as many as 10 million women in the United States suffer from PCOS. The syndrome does not discriminate and can be found in women of all races and ethnic groups throughout the world, although it tends to be more common in women of Mediterranean descent. PCOS affects women of all ages, from adolescence to menopause. Once a woman is diagnosed, she will need to manage the symptoms for the rest of her life.

Adolescent Females

Although the age of onset for PCOS symptoms varies, most women with PCOS can think back to their teenage years and remember a point in time when they started feeling "different" and wondering if something was wrong with them. Adolescent girls experience many of the same symptoms as adults—especially irregular or absent periods, unwanted hair, weight gain, and acne. For many adolescents, these physical changes seem to occur almost overnight. A young girl with PCOS can gain 30 or 40 pounds in just a few months even though she is exercising regularly and eating well. She also might start to suddenly notice more and more dark hair on her chin and upper lip, or maybe her face is beginning to break out despite her efforts to control it.

Adolescence can be a very difficult and emotional time for anyone. But for girls with PCOS, it can be even more difficult. They often feel isolated and confused. At an age when appearance is so important to them, girls with PCOS lose self-confidence as many of the symptoms start appearing. This feeling of confusion is only exacerbated since many girls have no one to talk to for information or encouragement. Girls often feel too embarrassed to seek help or even mention what is happening to them. Additionally, mothers, friends, or other close adults often don't understand what is happening either. It's important to find a knowledgeable physician who can perform appropriate hormone tests to determine whether a teen has PCOS.

Some of the newer research suggests that girls who begin to develop pubic hair early (usually before the age of 8), a condition known as *premature pubarche*, have many of the signs and symptoms of PCOS. These girls have both elevated insulin levels and elevated levels of DHEAS, a weak androgen. An elevated level of DHEAS is normally one of the first biochemical signs of awakening of the reproductive glands—in this case, the adrenal gland—after the long period of childhood inactivity. Throughout the rest of puberty, these girls produce excess testosterone and develop irregular periods consistent with PCOS. Thus, premature pubarche may be an early form of PCOS.

Women of Reproductive Age

Generally, a woman with PCOS will begin to experience menstrual irregularities within three to four years after her first period. After menstruation starts, a woman may have a few years of normal cycles until the symptoms of PCOS become evident. In some cases, women continue into their early 20s with normal cycles or no apparent PCOS symptoms before the symptoms begin.

Most women are diagnosed with PCOS during their 20s or 30s, although the reproductive years typically refer to the years between the late teens and the mid-40s. It is during this time that many women are trying to conceive. In fact, many women are not diagnosed until they seek medical treatment after being unable to get pregnant. Because PCOS is often diagnosed only after a woman has trouble conceiving, those women who are not trying to become pregnant often are not diagnosed. But PCOS is much more than a fertility issue. Women who for a variety of reasons are not currently trying to become pregnant will still benefit from treatment.

It is still unclear how PCOS changes as women age, especially as they enter their 30s and 40s. For some women, PCOS-related symptoms improve significantly as they get older. For others, the symptoms only worsen with age. Scientific research has not yet determined how factors such as weight loss, previous treatment with fertility drugs, or previous pregnancies or miscarriages affect women with PCOS over the course of their lives.

Menopausal Women

Menopause is the time in a woman's life when her menstrual cycle ends. This usually occurs around age 45 to 50. Symptoms of menopause include irregular periods, hot flashes, vaginal dryness, decline in sexual interest, mood changes, and night sweats. Menopause is usually determined after a woman has not had a period for one year or more. PCOS in menopausal women can go unnoticed since they always have irregular periods and often go long periods of time without menstruating at all.

Many women with PCOS believe that, since they have irregular periods, they won't go through menopause. However, this is not the case. It is important for menopausal women to seek treatment for both PCOS and menopausal symptoms.

Many women will take hormone replacement therapy to relieve menopausal symptoms and to decrease the risk of developing heart disease, osteoporosis, perhaps even Alzheimer's disease, stroke, and colon cancer. Because menopause causes a significant decrease in estrogen, many physicians prescribe estrogen. It can be given as a pill, as an implant (under the skin), or as a topical gel or patch. Some women, especially those with an intact uterus, are also given progesterone in addition to the estrogen. This helps protect the uterine lining against potentially harmful tissue changes, which can lead to endometrial cancer. The progesterone usually causes bleeding, similar to normal menstruation.

Unfortunately, hormone replacement therapy also comes with risks. These include a slightly increased risk of breast cancer and *thrombosis*, or blood clots. It is important to discuss both the benefits and risks with your doctor before you decide to start hormone replacement therapy. Also, make sure your health-care provider is familiar with PCOS and can help you select a treatment plan that will take into consideration the specific problems associated with PCOS.

Since many women are now living well past their 80s, the time spent post-menopausal can be thirty or more years. We know that women with PCOS are already at higher risk for developing diabetes, cardiovascular disease, and endometrial cancer. Because such risks only increase with age, treating PCOS during and after menopause can minimize the risk of developing these illnesses.

Why Diagnosis Is Difficult

PCOS is difficult to diagnose for several reasons.

First, many women do not report the symptoms of PCOS. Embarrassed about their symptoms, they do not talk openly with their physicians. Also, women often do not recognize that the various symptoms can be the result of a single cause.

Compounding the problem, many physicians lack current knowledge about diagnosing and treating PCOS. They may attribute PCOS to other causes, especially lifestyle factors such as too much stress or excess weight gain.

Furthermore, the term "polycystic ovary syndrome" itself can be misleading. The presence of cysts on the ovaries may or may not be a sign of PCOS. A single large cyst occurs naturally on the ovaries each month when the follicle containing an egg develops and ruptures. This cyst can reach a diameter of two to four inches but usually disappear with menses. Researchers estimate that 20 percent of women without PCOS have cysts on their ovaries. And approximately 30 percent of women with PCOS have "normal" ovaries with no cysts.

Of course, many women with PCOS do have multiple tiny cysts on their ovaries. In these cases, follicles begin to mature but never rupture to release the egg. As this process repeats month after month, multiple cysts form. The ovaries can become enlarged, taking on a thick, shiny, white coating, sometimes referred to as an "oyster shell." In women with many cysts, the cysts are said to resemble a "strings of pearls" lined up on the edge of the ovary.

It is important to get a diagnosis as soon as possible. Fortunately, there are many treatment options available to women with PCOS, once the condition is properly diagnosed.

Causes of PCOS

PCOS is the result of a hormonal imbalance, caused by a disorder in a woman's endocrine system. This system is made up of all the body's glands—pituitary, pineal, thyroid, parathyroid, thymus, adrenal, and pancreas. Hormones secreted by these glands control such things as growth, metabolism, and reproduction. In women with PCOS, this system is not working properly. Scientists believe there are several potential causes of this hormonal imbalance.

Insulin Resistance

For many years, PCOS was considered a direct result of high levels of male hormones in the body, although it was not understood exactly what caused these high levels. Researchers are now just beginning to understand the association between PCOS and the body's overproduction of insulin. Many women with PCOS have *hyperinsulinemia*, a higher than normal amount of insulin in their bodies. Hyperinsulinemia results from *insulin resistance.*

Insulin resistance results from the body not metabolizing sugar well. Let's take a closer look at the process, starting with the intake of food. As food enters your body, it is broken down into small components, including *glucose*, an important sugar that comes from carbohydrates. Glucose is a major source of quick energy for the body. When you eat foods high in carbohydrates, your body detects a rise in glucose and signals the pancreas to produce more insulin.

Together, glucose and insulin enter the bloodstream. The insulin fits into special "insulin receptors" in the cells. This allows the excess glucose to enter the cells and be used right away as energy or stored for future use. In the muscles and liver, glucose can be stored short-term as *glycogen.* In other tissues it can also be converted into fat for longer storage. To use an analogy, think of insulin as the key that unlocks the cell door so that excess glucose can enter and be converted to glycogen and stored for later use. When one has insulin resistance, it is as if the key no longer fits the lock. Consequently, the insulin is not able to fit into the insulin receptors, and excess glucose is not allowed to enter the cells. This causes a rise in both glucose and insulin levels in the blood.

In women with PCOS, these increased levels of glucose and insulin create an imbalance with other hormones. Subsequently, the body produces more male hormones and inhibits the ovaries from ovulating. This, in turn, causes the many PCOS-related symptoms. If left untreated, insulin resistance can lead to type II diabetes. Although insulin resistance is not found in every woman with PCOS, it is seen in many with PCOS, most prominently in those who are overweight.

Genetics

Researchers are finding that genetics seem to play a strong role in developing PCOS. However, this research is often difficult since most women, especially those from previous generations, were never "officially" diagnosed with PCOS. For example, there may be some women in your family who had difficulty getting pregnant but were eventually able to do so. Consequently, they may not think they had a problem with fertility. In addition, many of their other symptoms—weight gain, hair growth, and acne, for example—were either not serious or important enough to mention to their physicians.

Many leading researchers believe that PCOS is inherited. If you have a family history of adult-onset diabetes, infertility (or difficulty conceiving), obesity, or hirsutism (among women), then PCOS may run in your family. Similarly, inherited obesity can also increase the risk of developing the syndrome in those prone to developing it. Fatty tissues can produce estrogen, which can confuse the pituitary gland into secreting abnormal amounts of hormones, contributing to the overall endocrine problem.

Some scientists speculate that women with PCOS are born with either a faulty gene or set of genes that triggers abnormally high levels of male hormones. For example, if your sister has PCOS, there is a 50 percent chance that you will also have PCOS.

"There is no one officially diagnosed with PCOS in my family, but now that I have a better understanding of the condition, I see clearly that my mother has it and so did two of my dad's sisters and his mother. My dad is diabetic, as are several members of our extended family. No one takes me seriously when I try to get them to seek medical advice. They just count the diabetes and the heart conditions as the family curse," said Shelly, 29, a woman with PCOS. "They don't consider that PCOS could be part of the culprit in our family's medical problems."

Researchers believe that the genetics of PCOS can also be passed on to males, and they may experience some of the common symptoms. Male relatives of women with PCOS tend to be insulin resistant.

Other Theories

There are other theories about what causes PCOS, although most are not backed up by solid research. Some researchers and physicians have suggested that in utero (in the womb) experiences or a woman's emotional history may play a part as well.

One study suggests that the longer the duration of pregnancy—that is, the longer a pregnancy extends past 40 weeks—the greater the chance that PCOS will develop in the child later in life. Therefore, the researchers have suggested women not be allowed to go past 40 weeks of pregnancy. However, some physicians say that the child with PCOS would be more likely to have a mother with PCOS who would have had long cycles and late ovulation, making it seem as though the child was born post-term.

Another theory implies that internalized negative childhood messages about themselves contribute to women developing PCOS. Some women accept this suggestion. "I am a strong believer in the mind/body connection to any disorder," explained Michelle. "I don't think that PCOS is 'self-inflicted,' but I had a strong reaction to this theory. I realized that I had repressed sexual abuse from my childhood and my dad's disappointment over my not being a boy. After some self-reflection and a lot of crying and ranting and raving at my dear, patient husband, I started having really, really bad cramps and ended up shedding my whole, thick, built-up uterine lining as if my body was holding on to it along with all the guilt and shame I had been repressing. Doctors were amazed how 'overnight' this lining that they were considering dangerously thick was gone. I have learned a great deal about myself and how I internalize stress and how that affects my PCOS."

History of PCOS

This syndrome has baffled physicians for more than a century. In 1905, American gynecologists Dr. Irving Stein and Dr. Michael Leventhal were the first to officially describe PCOS. They both noticed a group of women who were experiencing similar symptoms—lack of periods, abnormal hair growth, obesity, and ovary enlargement caused by cysts. These doctors were the first to link the seemingly unrelated symptoms and give it a name, Stein-Leventhal syndrome. Later, the disorder was renamed polycystic ovary syndrome due to the polycystic ovaries that are found in many women who suffer from PCOS.

Today, in an attempt to better reflect the true nature of the condition, the syndrome is also called cystic ovaries, sclerocystic ovarian disease, functional ovarian hyperandrogenism (elevated levels of male hormones), hyperandrogenic chronic anovulation, and ovarian dysmetabolic syndrome.

Patients and physicians are beginning to see the need for a consistent name for the syndrome. A more accurate name would better describe the condition and prevent confusion in research, diagnosis, and treatment.

2

Living with PCOS Symptoms

Mornings were difficult for Rebecca, age 32. She was envious of other women she knew who were able to get ready for work in less than an hour. It always took Rebecca at least two hours to cover up all her PCOS symptoms. As she got out of the shower, she dried off in front of the mirror, preparing to do battle with her body.

First she had to painfully tweeze her extra facial hair, wincing as she pulled out each hair from above her lip and those around her chin, neck, and eyebrows. Close to tears, she trimmed excess hair from her forearms. Next, she rooted around her makeup bag for the special makeup she used to cover her acne. Using a thick concealer, she blended makeup along her jawline, feeling like a clown getting ready for a circus appearance.

Looking in the mirror, she sighed. She wished that for just one day she could look like everyone else. As if the extra weight wasn't enough to contend with, her appearance seemed so—well—freakish.

As Rebecca styled her hair, she realized her good fortune that she didn't have to worry about her hair thinning the way some women with PCOS did. Nevertheless, she was reluctant to wear her hair up because of the small skin tags on the back of her neck. Rebecca wasn't sure how noticeable they were to other people, but they embarrassed her.

Rebecca was afraid of doctors and didn't want to be reprimanded about her weight, but she knew it was time to do something. It was just too difficult to start every day like this.

Like many women with polycystic ovary syndrome, Rebecca combats symptoms that are cosmetic annoyances. However, the same hormonal imbalance that causes the cosmetic problems are also causing her irregular periods—one of the more serious symptoms of PCOS. In this chapter, we'll take a closer look at the symptoms of PCOS and examine ways of coping with them.

The Menstrual Cycle

PCOS is a leading cause of infertility. In fact, it may account for as many as half of all cases of infertility. Because women with PCOS often do not have regular menstrual cycles, they do not ovulate regularly, and their overall reproductive health is affected. To better understand how infertility occurs with PCOS, let's first examine how the normal menstrual cycle occurs.

Normal Menstrual Cycle

For most women, the menstrual cycle lasts approximately 28 days. The first day of menstruation, or bleeding, is considered Day 1. Bleeding usually ceases around Day 5. As bleeding stops, the hormone estrogen stimulates the lining of the uterus, the *endometrium*, to grow again in anticipation of a possible fertilized egg. From Day 14 until Day 28, the endometrium lining continues to grow from further stimulation of another hormone—progesterone. Progesterone is produced only if ovulation occurs.

On about Day 26 of a woman's cycle, if pregnancy does not occur, both the levels of estrogen and progesterone drop dramatically, which causes the endometrium lining to begin breaking down. The cycle is then completed, and bleeding begins again on Day 1. If a pregnancy does occur, the estrogen and progesterone levels remain elevated. This prepares and strengthens the endometrium to accept a fertilized egg, usually around day 21.

While all this is taking place in the uterus, by Day 28 of the cycle, just before bleeding occurs, the ovary is already working on developing a new *ovum*, or egg. By Day 6, just after bleeding has stopped, the new *follicle*, which contains the developing egg, is producing the estrogen necessary to promote the endometrial growth in the uterus. By Day 14 this egg bursts out of the follicle. This process is known as *ovulation* and signals the completion of the first half of the woman's cycle, which is known as the follicular phase.

High levels of three female hormones control the entire follicular phase, from follicle development to the release of an egg: *luteinizing hormone (LH), follicle-stimulating hormone (FSH),* and *estrogen.* LH and FSH are controlled by the pituitary gland, a small gland found in the brain. Under the influence of LH, the ruptured follicle, which once surrounded the egg, is transformed into a *corpus luteum*, a yellow mass in the ovary. FSH influences the maturation of the egg and its release from the ovary.

The corpus luteum produces high levels of estrogen and progesterone to encourage the growth of the endometrium, which will help sustain pregnancy until the placenta is formed and takes over. If pregnancy does not occur, the corpus luteum begins to break down around Day 26. This causes a drop in the levels of estrogen and progesterone, which in turn promotes the endometrium to be shed and bleeding to begin. If pregnancy does occur, the corpus luteum continues to secrete the hormones for the next 90 days.

This is an ideal menstrual cycle of 28 days. However, normal menstrual cycles can vary from a little more than 21 days up to 35 days. The part of the menstrual cycle that is most variable is the beginning, during the development of the preovulatory follicle, which can range from 7 to 21 days. The second half of the cycle after ovulation, called the *luteal phase,* is relatively fixed at 14 days.

Lack of a Menstrual Cycle in PCOS

As we can note from the description of normal ovulation, the menstrual cycle is perfectly synchronized. If a single hormone level is abnormal, many other hormones are affected and the entire cycle is disrupted. This is what happens to women affected by PCOS.

All women's bodies contain low levels of male hormones, or *androgens.* However, in women with PCOS, these levels are elevated. Even a small elevation in the hormones testosterone and DHEAS, can disrupt the menstrual cycle. They affect the feedback between the pituitary gland and the ovaries, leading to an abnormal production of LH and FSH—the hormones that stimulate the ovaries and promote ovulation. In women with PCOS, the level of LH is frequently, but not always, higher than usual, trying to start the cycle. As a result, the follicles never develop, but instead turn into small, pea-sized cysts on the ovaries.

The high levels of androgens also interfere with the FSH that is needed to trigger progesterone, which controls the shedding of the uterine lining and menstruation. Normally, the amounts of LH and FSH found in the body are roughly equal. In women with PCOS, the amount of LH can be two to three times or more the amount of FSH. Surprisingly, despite all this, estrogen levels are generally normal in women with PCOS. This is due largely to the high levels of androgens, which are converted by the body (and especially fat tissue) into estrogen, keeping the estrogen level within the normal range.

PCOS-related menstrual irregularities can be a vicious cycle of *anovulation*, or not ovulating, and *amenorrhea*, not menstruating. While some women with PCOS stop having menstrual cycles altogether, other women continue having their cycles. However, their cycles are usually highly irregular, and may not involve ovulation. This irregularity is called *oligomenorrhea*.

Abnormal hormone levels are the key factors in making it difficult to conceive. With irregular periods, or perhaps no periods for some women, there is no ovulation. No ovulation means no egg to fertilize, and consequently, no pregnancy can occur.

Hirsutism

One of the of the more difficult cosmetic symptoms of PCOS is *hirsutism*, excessive hair growth on the body. This unwanted hair usually grows above the lip or on the chin. It also occurs more thickly than usual on the limbs. There may also be hair on the chest or an extension of pubic hair on the abdomen and thighs. Such increased hair growth is usually noted in the late teen years and gradually increases as a woman gets older.

"The hirsutism is hard because it is such an outward, masculine sign," explained Beth, age 35. "For me, it became a problem at age 12. I started shaving after a particularly cruel comment from a junior high school boy. I have shaved ever since. I also remove hair on my chest, breasts, and stomach in addition to my armpits and legs. It even grows on my fingers."

There are a variety of methods for hair removal. You may wish to use one or a combination, depending on your needs and skin sensitivity.

Methods for Hair Removal

Medications

Several medications for hair removal can be prescribed. These include antiandrogenic medications, which counteract male hormones. In many cases, hair growth slows and hairs become thinner and less noticeable. It can take between six months and a year to notice much difference, and most medicines should be continued for several years. An important warning: many of these medications can cause birth defects if taken during pregnancy. Contraception or abstinence is the rule when these medications are used by women of reproductive age.

Spironolactone (Aldactone)

This medication directly fights the effects of androgens in the skin and can slowly reduce excessive hair growth, although it does not affect hair already present. This medication is often combined with an oral contraceptive. The contraceptive usually contains both estrogen and progesterone, hormones that may also help reduce excessive hair by stabilizing female hormone levels. Side effects include tender breasts. You should talk with your doctor about arranging a care plan that attempts these treatments in some reasonable combination or progression, with time limits set on each attempt.

"I've been on Aldactone for over two years and find it works really well for me," said Diana, age 22. "I used to wax my mustache, and now I pull only a few stray hairs with the tweezers once a month. The excess hair on other areas has also slowed to nearly nothing. The Aldactone also cleared up my complexion and knocked out the serious water retention problems I was having. If you use this drug, you have to stick with it. It takes a few months to really kick in, and all the symptoms come rushing back when you stop taking it."

Spironolactone may be associated with birth defects in male infants and should be avoided in women attempting pregnancy or who are pregnant.

Flutamide (Eulexin)

Another new drug that has proved helpful in treating hirsutism is flutamide (Eulexin). The drug manufacturer reports few side effects. However, some women may experience diarrhea, nausea, drowsiness, confusion, depression, anxiety, hypertension, loss of libido, anemia, elevated liver enzymes, rash, sensitivity to light, and hot flashes.

Cyproterone acetate

Cyproterone acetate blocks the male hormone dihydro-testosterone (DHT). It is often combined with an oral contraceptive and is effective for most women with hirsutism. Side effects, however, can include weight gain, depression, and loss of libido.

Vaniqua

Recently approved by the FDA, Vaniqua is the first prescription cream reported to reduce excessive facial hair in women. Studies show the medication helps most women and has no major side effects. The only side effects noticed in the research was a burning sensation and rash at the spot it was applied. The cream is applied to the face, like a moisturizer, twice a day. It works by blocking the enzyme that makes the hair follicles grow. It takes a few weeks for the cream to work. Vaniqua must be used regularly or hair growth will resume.

Oral Contraceptives

Oral contraceptives can help stabilize a woman's hormone levels, often reducing the growth of excess hair. Side effects include spotting (bleeding between periods), tender breasts, nausea, and headaches, especially in the first few months. Birth control pills are discussed in more detail in chapter 4.

Non-Medical Solutions for Hair Removal

Bleaching Hair

Bleaching doesn't remove the hair, but it makes the hair lighter and less obvious. Some women, however, do not like the way it looks when it grows back half blonde, half dark. For women with dark hair, it may look unusual to have blonde body hair. Others, with sensitive skin, may have a reaction to the bleaching chemicals or may dislike the odor of the chemicals in the removers.

Depilatory creams

Over-the-counter depilatory creams act like a chemical razor blade. (They are also available as lotions, gels, aerosols, and roll-ons.) A thick layer is applied to the skin for fifteen to thirty minutes, then wiped off, taking the hair with it. However, the creams can irritate the skin. It is important to read directions carefully because some creams are formulated only for certain areas of the body. Also, they should never be used on the eyebrows, or on broken or inflamed skin.

Shaving

Shaving is by far the most common method of hair removal. Shaving, twice a day if necessary, will prevent unsightly stubble. A clean razor with a sharp blade is essential for a safe and comfortable shave. Skin should never be shaved dry; wet hair is pliable and easier to cut. Contrary to popular opinion, shaving does not make the hair grow in more thickly or change the rate of hair growth.

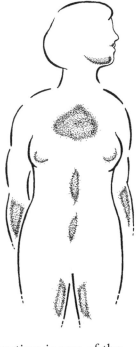

Hirsutism is one of the troublesome cosmetic symptoms of PCOS. Dark, excess hair often appears in the areas shown above—the upper lip, chest, arms, breasts, stomach, and thighs.

Tweezing and Waxing

Tweezing and waxing may be more painful than using a depilatory, but the results are longer lasting, and without strong chemical odors. However, tweezing is impractical for large areas

23

because it is a slow and painful process. It is mostly done for facial hair.

Waxing involves applying melted wax to the skin. After the wax hardens, it is stripped off, and hairs are pulled out by the roots. A small area should be tested before doing a large area. Waxing needs to be repeated every six weeks on the face, legs, underarms, and bikini areas. Waxes may be hot or cold, and may contain combinations of such ingredients as paraffin and beeswax, oils or fats, and a resin that makes the wax adhere to the skin. Waxing can be done in a beauty salon or at home. Some women have their own recipes for "sugaring," a homemade wax made with sugar and lemon juice. Some suggest waxing should only be done by an expert to limit the chance of infection.

Electrolysis

With professional electrolysis, a technician inserts a small probe along each hair, and a small electrical discharge destroys the hair follicle. This method may result in permanent hair loss, but it takes time. Only a small area is treated every few weeks. Electrolysis can be expensive if the affected area is extensive. Costs can range from $15 to $30 per fifteen minutes, and $25 to $50 for half an hour.

There are risks with the procedure. Scarring of the skin and electric shock can occur if the technician is unskilled. Other risks include infection which can be caused by an unsterilized needle. Many states require licensing, and you should seek a qualified individual to perform this procedure.

Let your electrologist know if you have any medical problems. Mention your PCOS and any medications you are taking. "My electrologist asks what medication I am on and writes a report on the hair growth for my doctor. She documents such things as new hair growth, how the treatments are keeping up with my hair growth, my mood, how my complexion looks, and whether she notices any weight gain or loss," explained Wanda, age 34. A good electrologist will also give you a short lesson on how hair grows.

According to Sara, age 35, "I've been going for electrolysis for twelve years. I started with my chin and neck. It took a long time to get it under control. Now the hair on my chin is gone, except for two, which take about six to seven weeks to grow back. The remaining hair on my neck is very light and blends in with my skin, except for several dark hairs that grow back every five to six weeks. The hair on my stomach bothers me, but not as much as the hair on my arms. So two years ago I started electrolysis on both forearms. The hair has thinned, but is still dark. Electroylsis isn't for everyone, and it does involve needles. It takes time and patience and can be expensive. But for me it is worth it."

Tips for Choosing an Electrologist

Ask friends for references. Call and ask for a free consultation. Ask if he/she is a certified public electrologist (CPE). Certification means the electrologist has gone through a voluntary testing program with the American Electrology Association, which also requires continuing education. Here are questions you should ask:

- What is the technician's education and experience?
- Are sterile, disposable needles used?
- Are all instruments sterilized after each use? Are approved sterilizers used?
- Does the technician wear gloves?

Finally, does the electrologist put you at ease? If you tried a treatment, did you feel the hairs being pulled? If so, let it be known. If he/she is unable to correct the problem, find another electrologist.

At-Home Electrolysis

At-home electrolysis machines have been on the market for about twenty years. Long term, the cost for one is less expensive than salon treatments. With these machines, tweezer epilators grasp the hair and send a low-level electric current down the shaft of the hair to the root. Reports vary on the effectiveness of these machines. They are not considered as effective as professional treatments.

Laser Therapy

New, long-wavelength lasers have been approved by the FDA for the removal of body hair. In recent years, laser hair removal has been advertised by more than 1,000 medical offices, salons, and day spas in the United States and Canada as the latest and greatest hair removal treatment. The FDA does not permit laser manufacturers to claim that laser treatment is permanent or painless, but they are permitted to advertise long-term results for hair removal. It is a faster route to the temporarily hairless look, but it is rarely permanent. Lasered hair often returns in three to six months. Laser treatment also carries a risk of scarring around the treated area.

Lasers must be used only by a licensed practitioner. The key to the effectiveness of the laser is proper adjustment of the pulse-width—the amount of time the laser is on and able to pass through the skin to reach the hair follicle. At the follicle level, the laser energy is absorbed and transformed into heat that disables the follicle. As a result, hair growth is impaired without affecting surrounding tissue. Each laser pulse treats about a one-half-inch area, which can contain ten or more hairs. The amount of time the treatment takes depends on the size of the area to be treated. Some lasers can treat an entire leg in half an hour and the upper lip in sixty seconds. Since some follicles can go dormant and produce hair at different times, several visits may be necessary for total treatment. Your physician will work with you to develop the optimal treatment strategy.

Most patients describe the treatment as feeling like a series of rubber band snaps to the skin. The majority of patients tolerate this sensation without anesthetics. However, for patient comfort, topical anesthetics or oral sedatives may be used. Within about thirty minutes of treatment, the skin may become pink or red and may feel like a mild sunburn for a day or so. Newer lasers are more efficient and cause less skin discoloration.

Pumice Stones

Some women have found the use of pumice stones to be a relatively painless way to remove unwanted hair. Hair is removed by lightly massaging the affected skin in a circular motion. The inexpensive pumice stones, found in natural foods stores, are said to work well. It is important to rinse the skin well afterwards to prevent infection. Apply a good moisturizer to avoid irritation because it can create a burn to the skin.

Acne

Adult acne is another particularly annoying problem for women with PCOS. It develops mostly on the face, especially the jawline, and on the chest and back. Acne forms when male hormones increase *sebum*, a combination of skin oils and old skin tissue, which clogs pores. Then, bacteria that thrive on sebum grow, resulting in pimples—whiteheads and blackheads.

Acne can be treated with both over-the-counter medications and several of the medications listed for the treatment of hirsutism. Since acne is caused by the same hormonal imbalance that causes hirsutism, antiandrogenic medications are frequently used to clear the skin.

If you decide to see a dermatologist about your acne, he/she might prescribe a topical treatment such as adapalene (Differin), or an antibiotic treatment such as tetracycline or erythromycin, or some combination of both. For more severe acne, the dermatologist might prescribe Accutane, a very potent oral medicine that helps to clear up the skin. Many of these medications used to treat acne, especially Accutane or Retin-A, cannot be used if you are pregnant, trying to become pregnant, or are nursing.

Women with PCOS experience varying degrees of success with treatments for acne. In addition to taking medications, women with PCOS are encouraged to spend extra time taking good care of their skin. The following skin care tips can help:

- Clean the skin gently but thoroughly with soap and water, removing all dirt or makeup. Wash as often as needed, at least daily and after exercising, to control oil. Use a clean washcloth every day to prevent bacterial reinfection.
- Use steam or a warm, moist compress to open clogged pores.
- Shampoo hair daily when possible. Use a dandruff shampoo if necessary.
- Comb or pull hair back to keep it out of the face.

- Use topical astringents to remove excess oil.

- Don't squeeze, scratch, pick, or rub lesions. These activities can increase skin damage. Wash your hands before and after caring for skin lesions to reduce the chance of infection.

- Don't rest your face on your hands. This irritates the skin of the face.

Weight Gain

Not all women with PCOS struggle with their weight, but many do. Those who do, gain weight for the same reason they have trouble losing weight—metabolic problems brought on by insulin resistance. As described earlier, a person who is insulin resistant eats food high in sugar (mainly carbohydrates, which are composed of sugar) but has difficulty breaking down the sugars. As a result, glucose and insulin levels increase, resulting in sudden weight gain. Furthermore, the increase in insulin also causes more male hormones to be produced, which also contributes to increased weight gain.

Another troublesome thing about insulin resistance is that once you eat carbohydrates and the insulin has finished its job of storing them, the body doesn't sit dormant waiting for more. Instead, it rushes a signal to the brain, giving out false hunger pains. Naturally, you eat more to satisfy your hunger, and the vicious cycle continues. And with each dose of carbohydrates you produce more and more insulin, causing hunger signals each time. This explains why you can become hungry one to three hours after eating a satisfying meal and why a sugary dessert can make you feel hungry again.

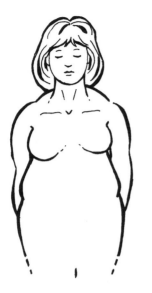

When PCOS women gain weight, the extra weight tends to accumulate in the waist, giving them an "apple shape." Here, the waist is larger than the hips.

Weight gain in PCOS women tends to result in an "apple-shaped" body, with the waist being thicker than the hips. This is more common of a male-pattern weight gain.

The weight gain in a woman without PCOS tends to result in a "pear-shaped" body, with the extra weight at the hips, buttocks, and thighs, while the waist remains thinner. Research shows that women with apple-shaped bodies tend to experience more health problems, including cardiovascular disease and diabetes.

Losing Weight

Losing weight is one of the best treatments for overweight women with PCOS. It helps to lower the level of insulin in the body. This, in turn, reduces the body's production of testosterone, alleviating many of the PCOS symptoms. Losing weight reduces the risk of cardiovascular disease and type II diabetes. It also boosts one's energy level and self-confidence. "When you have PCOS," explained Cori, 34, "you think more about how you feel about your body. Your relationship with your body is horrible."

Because the connection between PCOS and insulin resistance is so strong, many women have successfully lost weight by watching their carbohydrate intake, especially when other types of "diets" have failed. When fewer carbohydrates are coming in, your insulin and glucose levels drop and your body can actually burn fat for energy. This is what causes you to lose weight. "For the first time in my life I was successful at dieting with a low-carbohydrate food plan," said Diana, age 29. "I lost weight and I lost the cravings I had when my blood sugar dropped. When I go off 'low-carbing,' then my weight creeps back on, so I know this has to be a long-term commitment."

Increasingly, a low-carbohydrate diet is being touted as one of the best ways for women to lose weight. There are many popular low-carbohydrate diets. Some are more restrictive than others, so you might have to try several until you find one that you can stick to and is effective for you. For instance, you may decide to follow one of the popular low-carbohydrate, high-protein diets. Such diets recommend cutting your intake of carbohydrates to 30 grams or less a day. Once you have reached your goal weight, then you gradually increase your

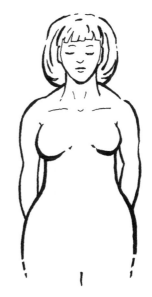

When women who do not have PCOS gain weight, the additional weight usually goes to the hips, giving them a "pear shape," in which the waist is still smaller than the hips.

carbohydrates until you stop losing weight. Women with diabetes, especially if they have co-existing vascular disease or renal impairment, are cautioned against low-carbohydrate and high-protein diets.

On the other hand, if you cannot totally give up carbohydrates, one of the less restrictive plans might be for you. Typically, no snacks are allowed, and two of your meals must be extremely low in carbohydrates. However, you are allowed one meal in which you can eat a moderate portion of carbohydrates. These diets are based on the theory that your body is primed on how much insulin to release based upon previous meals. So, with two meals of low carbohydrates and one meal of moderate carbohydrates, your body is tricked into releasing more insulin. Therefore, you store less fat and have steadier blood sugar levels.

Some women have successfully designed their own "moderate-carbohydrate" eating plans. You can create your own style of restricting your carbohydrate intake by simply eating mostly meats, eggs, cheeses, and vegetables. Foods high in carbohydrates are restricted as much as possible. Foods that tend to be high in carbohydrates include, but are not limited to: breads, cakes, cereal, chips, chocolate, cookies, crackers, fruit, ice cream, juice, pasta, potatoes, pretzels, rice, pie, popcorn, and sodas.

Note: it is not recommended that you avoid carbohydrates altogether. Everyone needs to eat some carbohydrates. It is extremely important when designing your own eating plan to make sure the meals are balanced. This means you should eat a variety of nutritious foods, balancing the carbohydrates with vegetables and foods high in protein. In addition, the carbohydrates should not all come from the "junk food" category—chips, chocolate, cookies, ice cream, and the like. Fortunately, there are many low- or moderate-carbohydrate cookbooks now available that can help you design a well- balanced menu.

Another important part of watching your carbohydrate intake is paying particular attention to serving size. Although the food "pyramid," recommended by the Food and Drug Administration, suggests that Americans eat six to eleven servings of breads and grains (foods high in carbohydrates), most people eat far much more than this based on their lack of knowledge of appropriate serving sizes. Examples of serving sizes for breads and grains include one slice of bread, one ounce of cereal, and a half cup of rice or pasta. Therefore, one bagel consists of two servings, one for each half. The same can be said for a sandwich—one serving for each slice of bread. Furthermore, if you decide to eat pasta, you might very well be eating three or four servings of carbohydrates instead of the recommended half-cup for a single serving. As you can see, it is easy for the typical person to surpass the recommended six to eleven servings from this food group. For women with PCOS, this lack of knowledge about serving sizes for carbohydrates can lead to significant increases in insulin levels.

Before you decide to try any new eating plan, it is important to talk to your health-care professional. He/she can then thoroughly assess your health status and help direct you toward a plan that will meet your specific needs.

Exercise

Exercise is an essential treatment for women with PCOS. It can help women in several ways. Exercise plays an important part in weight loss. It is also proven to help achieve proper insulin levels, which, in turn, affect hormone levels. Exercise helps you feel good about your body and gives you a sense of accomplishment.

Cori, who jogs every other day and weight trains on alternate days, knows that not all women with PCOS are able or willing to jog three miles at a time. "We all just need to move, whether it is yoga or water aerobics or walking. Exercising has changed my life. "

Baldness and Thinning Hair

In some women, male-pattern hair loss, or *androgenic alopecia,* is an unwelcome reminder of living with PCOS. This may be due to an increase in androgens, or male hormones. In alopecia, hairs become smaller and smaller during each growth phase. Hair usually thins the most on the top of the head, the part of the scalp that is most androgen sensitive. Frontal balding and hairline recession is seen only in the most severe cases.

Medications for Baldness or Thinning Hair

Minoxidil (Rogaine)

Minoxidil (Rogaine) is the most widely recommended treatment for male-pattern baldness. The drug appears to work by gradually enlarging and lengthening hair follicles that have been gradually shrinking. The growth phase may also be extended, giving the hairs an opportunity to lengthen before they fall out. It takes about three to four months of use to see evidence of any regrowth and up to six months to determine whether minoxidil will be beneficial.

One fact of life with minoxidil: it must be used continually. Once discontinued, any new hair growth will be lost. Minoxidil may exceed the budgets of some individuals; however, a generic version is less expensive. Because these drugs are considered cosmetic treatments, their cost is usually not covered by health insurance.

Retin-A / Tretinoin

Retin-A is used as a topical treatment for acne and other skin disorders. A vitamin-A ointment, it can be used alone or in combination with minoxidil. Retin-A has been known to produce moderate to good hair growth in individuals with male-pattern baldness and *alopecia areata*, total baldness. If a combination is used, it is suggested that minoxidil be applied in the morning and the Retin-A gel in the evening to reduce the problem of skin sensitivity to sunlight. In addition to increased sun sensitivity, the side effects of Retin-A can include blistering and altered pigmentation. Many dermatologists also recommend using tretinoin, another topical vitamin-A preparation, in combination with minoxidil to enhance minoxidil's effect. These medications should not be used by pregnant women.

Depression

Understanding depression as a symptom of PCOS is still relatively new, especially because it can be difficult to know whether depression is a symptom of PCOS or whether the PCOS symptoms such as weight gain and infertility cause the depression. Most researchers do agree that a woman's physiology, which is so closely related to hormone fluctuations, is an important key to understanding depression. Hormones influence our behavior as well as our health in complex ways still not completely understood by medical science.

Given the importance of depression as a possible symptom, it is discussed more fully in chapter 8.

Skin Abnormalities

Skin Tags

Skin abnormalities in women with PCOS can take a variety of forms. Skin tags, or *acrochordons*, are teardrop-shaped pieces of skin usually found in the armpits or around the neck. They are often about the size of a pinhead but can be as large as a raisin. Skin tags are common, benign growths that occur most often after midlife. They are usually painless, except for occasional irritation from rubbing by clothing or other friction, and do not grow or change. Their origin is unknown. They are thought to be a symptom of insulin resistance and can be removed by a physician. Insurance will usually pay for the procedure if you explain to the physician that the condition is irritated by wearing jewelry or your bra strap. This way it will not be billed as a cosmetic procedure.

"I have those Rice Krispy-looking things two or three at a time," explained Michelle, age 38. "One time I tied dental floss around one and tightened it every day until it fell off, but then it got infected and I still had to go to the doctor. I heard of another woman who just cut it off, but her armpit was swollen for a week. Now, my dermatologist removes them. This is the safe way to handle skin tags."

"Dirty" Skin

Another unusual skin problem is *acanthosis nigricans*, a disorder that causes light-brown-to-black, velvety, rough areas on the back and sides of the neck. Women say that their skin looks "dirty." The condition can also occur under the arms and in the groin. Acanthosis nigricans may begin at any age.

When acanthosis nigricans develops, a medical evaluation should be done to determine whether the patient has an endocrine gland disorder, such as an insulin-secreting tumor. Prescriptions that may provide some improvement for this condition include insulin sensitizers to lower insulin levels, or topical solutions such as Retin-A, alpha hydroxy acid, and salicylic acid.

Migraines

Cindy, age 34, remembers her first migraine at 15. "The pain was intense and I felt nausea and a great sensitivity to light. I sat in a dark room for an hour and it finally passed."

The pain of a classic migraine headache is described as intense, throbbing, or pounding and is felt in the forehead, temple, ear, jaw, or around the eye. The migraine starts on one side of the head but may eventually spread to the other side. Other symptoms include nausea and at times disturbed vision. An attack can last a few hours or up to one to two pain-wracked days. There are some indications that women with PCOS may be predisposed to migraines.

Scientists report that some women with migraines who take birth control pills experience more frequent and severe attacks. However, a small percentage of women have fewer and less severe migraine headaches when they take birth control pills. Investigators around the world are studying hormonal changes in women with migraines in the hope of identifying the specific ways that these naturally occurring chemicals cause headaches.

For infrequent migraines, medications can be taken at the first sign of a headache to stop it or to at least ease the pain. People who get occasional, mild migraines may benefit by taking aspirin or acetaminophen at the start of an attack. Aspirin raises a person's tolerance to pain and also discourages the clumping of blood platelets. Small amounts of caffeine may be useful if taken in the early stages of a migraine. But for most migraine sufferers, those who get moderate to severe headaches, stronger drugs may be necessary to control the pain. If you suffer from migraines, discuss your treatment options with your physician.

A number of alternative therapies have achieved some success for women with migraines. Professional massage, chiropractic, or osteopathic manipulation can be done to enhance circulation and relax the muscles. Acupuncture, hypnosis, and aromatherapy are less documented, although some women find them helpful. Exercising is also thought to help by releasing *endorphins*, which offer pain relief. Tai chi and yoga may also be beneficial.

Other Symptoms

Because the symptoms of PCOS can vary widely, it can be difficult to exclude or include many other symptoms as a part of the diagnosis. Research is being done to examine other possible symptoms of PCOS such as sleep apnea, retinopathy, and irritable bowel syndrome. There may very well be more common symptoms of PCOS discovered as new studies are completed and women with PCOS continue talking and gathering their own evidence.

3

Getting a Diagnosis

Twenty-five-year-old Nicole had read a short article about PCOS in a popular woman's magazine. She seemed to have many of the symptoms—being overweight, unwanted hair, and no periods. Nicole was sure she had PCOS. Unfortunately, she did not want to see a doctor to confirm this diagnosis. She had always hated going to the doctor. To make matters worse, Nicole had just moved to a new city three months ago, and she didn't even want to think about finding a new gynecologist. Further, she thought by going to the doctor, she would only be subjected to numerous uncomfortable tests, not to mention she would be embarrassed to discuss her symptoms and concerns with a doctor she didn't know.

Her previous doctor, whom she had seen since she was 18, never seemed interested in her concerns. She knew PCOS was not curable, so what could a physician do? Nicole decided to put off seeing a doctor.

One year later, she finally decided to see a new doctor after a friend recommended a gynecologist and raved about how nice and caring this doctor was. Still a little nervous about possibly having PCOS, Nicole decided to give it a try. The doctor asked some good questions about Nicole's personal and family health history and also explained to Nicole that although her symptoms indicated she had PCOS, there was no way to confirm the diagnosis without some simple tests. Nicole agreed to have an ultrasound and some blood tests to measure hormone levels.

A few days later, when the ultrasound and blood work were completed, the doctor called Nicole back to her office. She confirmed that Nicole had PCOS. Nicole was relieved to finally understand her problem and begin treatment for it. Together, she and her doctor discussed various treatment options. Now Nicole only wishes she had seen a doctor sooner.

Choosing a Physician

Women with PCOS often complain that finding a good health-care provider can be tough. Although many physicians are not knowledgeable about PCOS, the situation is improving. Physicians are becoming more knowledgeable about this topic, and women with PCOS are becoming more informed and aggressive in their search for treatment.

Many women have seen several doctors before finding the right one. There are several ways to find a good physician to manage your PCOS. First of all, you can contact the Polycystic Ovarian Syndrome Association (PCOSA). This organization maintains a state-by-state listing of member physicians who are interested in treating women with PCOS. Also, you can contact RESOLVE, an international support group that focuses on women and couples experiencing infertility, for a listing of physicians in your area who specialize in infertility issues. Other possible sources for finding a physician include a local PCOSA chapter, your primary care provider, a hospital network's referral services, insurance companies, or professional associations such as the American Society of Reproductive Medicine and the Endocrine Society. When selecting a physician, remember to take into consideration your health insurance plan and proximity to specialists. Managing PCOS is an ongoing process and may require many visits to your doctor's office.

When selecting a physician, consider asking the following questions:

- **How soon can an appointment be scheduled?** Most women with PCOS have already seen several doctors who have not provided them with a proper diagnosis for their symptoms. Therefore, many of these women are eager to see a knowledgeable physician and might find it difficult to wait several months for an appointment. Also, find out how long you will have to wait to see the doctor again for follow-up care. Find out if your doctor will be available for telephone consults if you end up having any further questions about your diagnosis or treatment.

- **Is there a physician in the practice who specializes in PCOS?** Ask the physician how many women with PCOS he/she has treated and how he/she typically treats it. This will give you a good idea as to the physician's current experience in helping women overcome PCOS symptoms.

- **What is the physician's background?** Ask about education, experience, and years in practice. Being diagnosed and treated for PCOS can be very emotional, so try to select a physician with whom you will feel comfortable.

- **How does the physician typically diagnose and treat PCOS?** Look for a physician who considers personal and family history as well as blood tests and ultrasounds when diagnosing PCOS. Decide how you would like to progress in your treatment of PCOS. If you are trying to become pregnant, do you want to be aggressive or do you prefer to take it slow? Once you have made a decision, select a physician who will meet your expectations.

- **Does the physician test for insulin problems and recommend treatment to improve them?** Current research is stressing the link between PCOS and insulin resistance. It is important to make sure that your physician is aware of this research and is incorporating this new information in how he/she addresses PCOS.

- **Does the health-care provider integrate or recommend natural or dietary therapies?** Since not every therapy works for every woman, some women are looking for a more holistic approach. More and more evidence is showing the importance of nutrition and exercise in managing PCOS. If this type of treatment interests you, make sure you select a physician who supports your views.

Most women first turn to their obstetrician/gynecologist (OB/GYN) or primary care physician when looking for a diagnosis. Some women with PCOS end up seeing several OB/GYNs before they find one with whom they feel comfortable. The key is to not give up.

Since many women see nurse practitioners, physician assistants, or certified nurse-midwives for gynecological care, these health-care providers are becoming more and more knowledgeable about PCOS and are often able to make an accurate diagnosis. However, they are often more limited than physicians in their ability to provide a wide range of treatments.

Many women with PCOS, especially those who are trying to become pregnant, decide to see a specialist called a *reproductive endocrinologist (RE)*. REs focus on women or couples who are having difficulty conceiving, including those with PCOS. This is covered in more detail in chapter 7.

If you are not trying to get pregnant and still would like to see a specialist, you might want to try a *general endocrinologist*, a physician who specializes in all hormonal disorders, or a reproductive endocrinologist whose practice is not limited to infertility.

Since PCOS can encompass a wide range of symptoms, it is possible that you will see a number of different types of health-care providers. For example, you may see a cardiologist for your high cholesterol and a dermatologist for acne. These physicians may want to prescribe different medications that treat each symptom individually. Therefore, it is important to make all your health-care providers aware that you have PCOS and explain what medications you are taking. It will also be your responsibility, as the patient, to find health-care providers who will be aware of treating your PCOS completely and not each symptom individually.

Diagnostic Testing

PCOS is greatly underdiagnosed. It's estimated that only about 10 percent of women with the syndrome have received a diagnosis. PCOS cannot be self-diagnosed. Nor can it be diagnosed by a physician solely based on reported symptoms. Taking symptoms and family history into consideration, a physician can diagnose PCOS only through a series of diagnostic tests. These include blood tests, which measure hormone levels, and a transvaginal ultrasound, which examines the uterus and ovaries.

Testing Hormone Levels

Assessing hormone levels serves two purposes. First of all, it helps confirm the diagnosis. Secondly, it can rule out other illnesses that might be causing the symptoms. Other medical problems can create symptoms similar to those of PCOS; these include menopause, pituitary tumors, and problems with adrenal or thyroid glands. When doctors are considering a diagnosis of PCOS, they will draw blood to test the levels of various hormones, including those listed below.

Luteinizing Hormone (LH)
and Follicle-Stimulating Hormone (FSH) Levels

LH and FSH are secreted by the pituitary gland in the brain. These hormones encourage ovulation. At the beginning of the menstrual cycle, LH and FSH levels are usually about equal. However, roughly twenty-four hours before ovulation occurs, the amount of LH increases significantly. This surge in LH is what causes the egg to be released from the ovary. Once the egg is released by the ovary, the LH level goes back down to its original pre-surge level.

Many women with PCOS already have an elevated LH level, so the amounts of LH and FSH at the beginning of the cycle are no longer equal. Although some women with PCOS still have LH and FSH levels that appear within the "normal" range, their LH level is often two or three times or more than that of the FSH level. This situation is called an *elevated LH to FSH ratio*. Because the amounts of LH and FSH should be very similar, this change in the LH to FSH ratio is enough to disrupt ovulation.

Testosterone Level

All women have some amount of the male hormone testosterone in their bodies. To determine the amounts of the hormone present, your doctor may measure your *total testosterone*, the total amount circulating in your body. He/she may also measure your *free testosterone*, the amount circulating freely in your body. Free testosterone significantly contributes to such symptoms as excessive hair growth, baldness, and acne. Women with PCOS often have an increased level of both total testosterone and free testosterone. Some women with PCOS have total testosterone levels that are still within the "normal" range, although often on the high end of "normal." However, even a slight increase in testosterone in a woman's body (even if it is still within the "normal range) can suppress normal menstruation and ovulation and lead to other PCOS-related symptoms.

DHEAS Level

DHEAS or *dehydroepiandrosterone* sulfate is another male hormone that is found in all women. It is secreted by the adrenal gland. Women with PCOS often have elevated DHEAS levels. Similar to the testosterone levels, DHEAS levels that appear within the higher limits of the "normal" range are common among PCOS women. However, depending on the individual, even a minor increase in DHEAS, especially in conjunction with an increase in testosterone, can contribute to PCOS-related symptoms.

Prolactin Level

Prolactin is the hormone that stimulates and sustains milk production in nursing mothers. Prolactin levels are usually normal in women with PCOS. However, some PCOS women have a slightly elevated level of prolactin, or *hyperprolactinemia*, which tells the body to produce milk. It can sometimes cause a white discharge from the breasts, even if you are not pregnant. It is important to check for high prolactin levels in order to rule out other problems, such as a pituitary tumor, that might be causing symptoms similar to those caused by PCOS.

Androstenedione (ANDRO) Level

ANDRO is another male hormone that is produced by the ovaries and adrenal glands. It is more potent than DHEAS, but signifcantly less potent than testosterone. Sometimes high levels can affect estrogen and testosterone levels, which in turn can contribute to PCOS-related symptoms.

Progesterone Level

Progesterone is produced by the corpus luteum after ovulation occurs. It helps to prepare the uterine lining for pregnancy. Testing levels of this hormone is especially important. Sometimes women with PCOS can show signs that ovulation is occurring; however, when the progesterone test is done, it shows that ovulation did not occur. If this happens, your body is producing a follicle and preparing you to ovulate, but for some reason the egg is not being released from the ovary. In addition, low progesterone levels may tell your doctor that your body is not producing enough progesterone on its own to sustain a pregnancy even if the egg is being released. All this information can help your physician possibly adjust fertility medications for the next cycle to encourage the release of the egg and help sustain a pregnancy.

Estrogen Level

Estrogen is the female hormone that is secreted mainly by the ovaries and in small quantities by the adrenal glands. The most active estrogen in the body is called *estradiol*. A sufficient amount of estrogen is needed to work with progesterone to promote menstruation. Most women with PCOS are surprised to find that their estrogen levels fall within the normal range. This may be due to the fact that the high levels of androgens found in women with PCOS can sometimes be converted to estrogen.

Thyroid-Stimulating Hormone Level (TSH)

Thyroid-stimulating Hormone (TSH) is produced by the thyroid gland in the neck. Women with PCOS usually have normal TSH levels. TSH is checked to rule out other problems, such as an underactive or overactive thyroid, which often causes irregular or absent periods and no ovulation.

Glucose Level for Insulin Resistance

There are two tests for insulin resistance and diabetes. One is the *fasting plasma glucose (FPG) test*, a simple blood test taken after eight hours of fasting. It measures the levels of sugars in the blood. Elevated levels indicate insulin resistance. The test is not always reliable. If a person has normal levels but has symptoms of diabetes and a family history or other risk factors, diabetes should not be ruled out, and other tests should be performed.

The *glucose tolerance test* is more sophisticated. It includes an FPG test, along with a blood test, which is taken two hours after drinking a glucose solution. Normally, blood sugar increases modestly after drinking the glucose beverage and decreases after two hours. In the diabetic, the initial increase is excessive and the level remains high.

Hormone Ranges Vary

It is important to remember that hormone levels among women can vary greatly, and the variations mean that women don't always have the same symptoms. It is also important to mention that the "normal" ranges can vary since each lab sets its own "normal" values. Some women have hormone levels that appear within the "normal" range but still suffer from symptoms and still might have PCOS. This is especially true with testosterone, DHEAS, and LH levels. Even small changes in these hormone levels can cause PCOS symptoms.

The table of "normal" hormone values is a tool you can use with your physician to discuss your hormone levels and what they mean. Seek the advice of a specialist if you have a testosterone level greater than 40 ng/ml, a DHEAS level greater than 200 ug/dl, or an LH level that is two or three times that of your FSH level. LH and FSH levels should be roughly equal during the early part of the menstrual cycle. Note that even small abnormalities in hormone levels can cause PCOS symptoms.

Hormone Values

Normal Range
FSH

Cycle Day 3: 3-20 mIU/ml
Cycle Day 10: 19-28 mIU/ml
(about twice Day 3 level)

PCOS Range

Most often FSH levels fall within the normal range. FSH and LH levels should be roughly equal at Cycle Day 3.

Normal Range	PCOS Range
LH	
Cycle Day 3: 5-20 mlU/ml "Surge" Day: 25-40 mlU/ml	For Cycle Day 3, sometimes LH levels fall within the normal range; however, LH is often elevated making it two or three times greater than the FSH level. For "Surge" Day, often women with PCOS are unable to detect a surge of LH during their cycle, meaning that they are not ovulating.
Estrogen or Estradiol	
Cycle Day 3: 25-75 pg/ml	Should be within normal range.
Progesterone	
Cycle Day 21 (or 7 days post ovulation): Greater than 14 ng/ml	If ovulation is occurring, should be within the normal range.
Prolactin	
Less than 25 ng/ml	For most, should be within the normal range. For some, slightly elevated prolactin levels, falling within the 25-40 ng/ml range.
TSH	
0.4-5.0 uIU/ml	Should be within the normal range.
Total Testosterone	
6.0-86 ng/dl	Usually greater than 40 ng/dl.
Free Testosterone	
Less than 5 pg/ml	Usually elevated.
DHEAS	

Normal Range	PCOS Range
35-430 ug/dl	Usually greater than 200 ug/dl.

ANDRO

0.7-3.1 ng/ml	Usually elevated

Fasting Plasma Glucose

Less than 110 mg/dl	Insulin Resistant (at-risk for developing diabetes): 110-126 mg/dl
	Type II Diabetes: Greater than 126 mg/dl

Glucose Tolerance Test with Insulin

Normal Levels	PCOS Levels
Fasting: Glucose: <126 mg/dl Insulin: < 10 mIU/ml	*Fasting:* Insulin levels above 10mIU/ml may indicate insulin resistance. Glucose levels of more than 126 mg/dl indicates type 2 diabetes.
After one hour: Glucose <140 mg/dl	*After one hour:* Insulin levels of more than 4.5 times that of the fasting levels may indicate insulin resistance. Glucose levels of 140-199 mg/dl indicate risk for type 2 diabetes. Glucose levels of more than 200 mg/dl indicates type 2 diabetes.

Checking Cholesterol Level

Cholesterol is not a hormone. Rather, it is a waxy, fat-like substance found in every cell. It is normally used by the body to form cell membranes and certain hormones. Cholesterol is carried throughout the body by *lipoproteins*. There are two types of lipoproteins: *low-density lipoproteins (LDL)*, the so-called bad cholesterol, and *high-density lipoproteins (HDL)*, the so-called good cholesterol. LDL can mix with other substances, forming *plaque*, which builds up in artery walls and causes dangerous blockages. HDL removes cholesterol from the blood and carries it to the liver to be metabolized. *Triglycerides*, another component of cholesterol, tend to be high in women with PCOS, further contributing to the risk of heart disease.

Researchers are beginning to notice a connection between PCOS and high cholesterol levels. Therefore, some physicians may want to check your cholesterol levels. Women with PCOS have a greater tendency to have high cholesterol, a major risk factor for developing heart disease. Even if your physician does not check your cholesterol levels when diagnosing PCOS, it is a good idea to have these levels checked periodically to prevent heart disease.

It is important to check all three components of cholesterol, plus the *total cholesterol* in the body. The following measurements show normal and undesirable cholesterol levels.

LDL Cholesterol (mg/dl)
> Desirable: less than 130
> Borderline-high: 130-159
> High: greater than 160

HDL Cholesterol (mg/dl)
> Greater than 35 is acceptable
> Less than 35 creates risk factor

Triglycerides (mg/dl)
> Desirable: less than 200, high: greater than 400

Total Cholesterol (mg/dl)
> Desirable: less than 240
> Borderline-high: 200-239
> High: greater than 240

Transvaginal Ultrasound

Another important tool for diagnosing PCOS is the *transvaginal ultrasound.* This method uses sound waves to produce images of your reproductive organs. In this procedure, the doctor inserts a hand-held, cylinder-shaped instrument called a *transducer* into your vagina. Your doctor will move the transducer within your vagina to measure your ovaries to see if they are enlarged, to determine whether you have any cysts, and to view your endometrium—the lining of your uterus. For most women, the transvaginal ultrasound only takes a few minutes and is no more painful or uncomfortable than a regular pelvic exam.

Personal and Family History

To fully understand your medical history and how it relates to PCOS, your physician should take a thorough personal and family history. You will likely be asked the following things about your menstrual history:

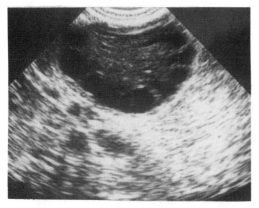

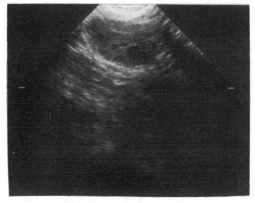

Ultrasound of a Cystic Ovary

The ovary is the darker mass toward the top of the photo. Note how cysts cluster around the edge of the ovary, giving it a black "pearl necklace" appearance.

Ultrasound of Normal Ovary

The normal ovary has a more consistent appearance, with only scattered follicles, as indicated by the small follicle in the lower right-hand edge of the ovary.

- Age at first period
- Length of menstrual cycle
- Regularity of menstrual cycle
- How your periods have changed over time
- How much bleeding is present during a cycle
- Period-related symptoms—pain, bloating, headaches

In addition, you will be asked about your reproductive history:
- Birth control methods used in the past
- Length of time you have been trying to get pregnant
- Number of pregnancies

- Number of miscarriages and/or abortions
- Menstrual irregularities or infertility issues experienced by your mother, sisters, or aunts

While your physician is collecting this information, it's important that you are completely honest. You will also want to discuss in detail with your physician all the symptoms that you have been experiencing, even if you are embarrassed or don't think they relate to PCOS. Also, let your physician know if you have a family history of infertility, diabetes, heart disease, stroke, or cancer. Once a diagnosis is obtained, you and your physician can work together to decide on your treatment goals.

4

Medical Treatments

Rene, 29, was delighted to begin successful treatment for PCOS. She wanted to start a family, but PCOS had prevented her from ovulating regularly. Previous treatments, prescribed by other doctors, had been unsuccessful. Only after finding a new gynecologist did she feel hopeful. It had been just six months since she had started seeing the physician, who had been recommended by a woman in her PCOS support group. This doctor was well informed about PCOS and had listened to Rene's list of symptoms and asked careful questions.

Since beginning the new treatment plan, Rene was making progress. Although she wasn't pregnant yet, for the first time ever, she had a couple of normal menstrual cycles. At last, Rene felt that her medical treatment was working.

Women's personal goals vary when they are considering medical therapy for PCOS. For some women, getting pregnant may be the ultimate goal. For others, addressing cosmetic symptoms like hirsutism may be high on the list. What matters most to you? List the top three aspects of PCOS that you would like to see change. Take the list to your health-care provider and discuss it. When you see a health-care provider with clear goals in mind, it is more likely that your treatment plan will work.

Benefits of Treatment for PCOS

The benefits of treatment are numerous. PCOS can be treated effectively with a variety of medications. For example, many women, with the help of drug therapy, can successfully carry a pregnancy to term. Other medications can restore a normal menstrual cycle. As mentioned earlier, without a normal menstrual cycle, women with PCOS are at risk for such diseases as endometrial cancer and cardiovascular disease. A woman with PCOS is seven times more likely to develop cardiovascular disease and has a 40 percent chance of developing diabetes. There aren't yet cures for PCOS, but with education and treatment, the risks can be minimized.

Drugs Commonly Prescribed for PCOS

Many medications are used to treat PCOS. A number of these can have multiple benefits. For example, a birth control pill may help a woman resume a regular period and also help reduce excess hair growth. These improvements occur as a result of changes in hormonal levels. Yet there is no uniform pill or prescription for everyone. Each woman's symptoms vary, and she may respond differently to a drug. Accordingly, you and your physician may need to work at finding the right drug or combination of drugs that most help you.

In an earlier chapter, we discussed medications often used to treat the cosmetic symptoms of PCOS. In this chapter, we'll discuss some of the drugs that are commonly prescribed to treat the "internal" problems. You'll notice that the benefits of some of the drugs cross categories and are useful in both situations.

Insulin Sensitizers

The newer treatments for PCOS aim at the root cause— elevated insulin levels. Insulin sensitizers are intended to help the body begin to effectively process insulin again. These medications were originally prescribed to people with type II diabetes but have also been shown to successfully treat women with PCOS who have insulin resistance.

Let's use the door-and-key analogy again. Insulin sensitizers help the body rediscover the key to unlock the cell doors, allowing the entry and storage of excess glucose. As insulin and glucose levels return to normal, the ovary resumes normal function, and many of the other hormones return to a more appropriate level. In turn, many PCOS symptoms diminish. For many women, insulin sensitizers restore menstrual cycles and alleviate such symptoms as hair growth on the body, thinning hair, acne, and excess weight. Insulin sensitizers lower the risk of cardiovascular disease and diabetes. These medications may also cause insulin-resistant women to start ovulating again.

If you are taking insulin sensitizers, report any changes in your monthly cycle to your doctor. In addition, let your health-care provider know if you are trying to become pregnant, are already pregnant, or are breast-feeding. Side effects of insulin sensitizers are rare. Although these medications lower elevated blood sugar levels in people with diabetes, when given to women with high insulin levels, they *only* lower insulin levels. Blood sugar levels will not change; therefore, women will not experience episodes of "low blood sugar."

Because research has indicated that some insulin sensitizers might cause liver problems, your physician should monitor your liver function by conducting periodic blood tests as a precaution if any of the medications are prescribed for you.

Call your health-care provider right away if you develop nausea, vomiting, stomach pain, loss of energy or appetite, dark urine, or jaundice (yellow coloring of the eyes and skin). These may be symptoms of potential liver problems.

Metformin (Glucophage)

One insulin sensitizer, *metformin* whose brand name is *Glucophage,* seems to alliviate PCOS symptoms for many. It is not approved by the FDA to treat PCOS, but is approved as a treatment for diabetes; it has been found to lower insulin levels.

"I am so glad I decided to take it," said Julie, 38. "Since being on metformin, my outlook on life in general has greatly improved. I am not tired all the time, and most importantly, I enjoy playing with my kids again. I had a few gastro side effects—a little diarrhea and a little nausea. I even lost weight without changing my eating habits, although I am not sure if that has anything to do with the nausea."

Approximately 30 percent of patients started on Glucophage will experience gastrointestinal symptoms: diarrhea, nausea, vomiting, abdominal bloating, flatulence, and loss of appetite. These symptoms are usually temporary (one to four weeks) and will disappear during continued therapy. It is advisable for new patients to initiate therapy slowly to minimize the gastrointestinal side effects.

"As a nurse, I can tell you that almost everyone who goes on this develops GI (gastrointestinal) symptoms to some degree," said Julie. "My endocrinologist said, 'Take this with food to avoid the GI upset.' I found I did best by taking the metformin halfway through the meal. The food 'cushions' the pill, and the GI upset is lessened or in many cases eliminated. You may have diarrhea or nausea regardless of what you do for approximately seven days minimally, so don't give up if that happens. Keep doing it and you'll see a significant improvement."

According to some women, metformin's side effects may also include hair loss, however. This may prove too much for women already struggling with thinning hair. The drug has also been associated with a rare condition called *lactic* acidosis in which too much lactic acid, byproducts of carbohydrate metabolism, builds up in the blood stream; it is potentially life threatening. However, reported cases have occurred primarily in diabetic patients with severe renal (kidney) insufficiency.

Pioglitazone (ACTOS)

Another insulin sensitizer, *pioglitazone*, brand name ACTOS, may normalize other hormones such as testosterone and LH. Another added benefit seen with pioglitazone is a reduction in the levels of triglycerides, fat-carrying molecules, which are one component of cholesterol. There were no notable side effects in clinical trials.

Rosiglitazone (Avandia)

This drug works in a fashion similar to ACTOS by improving insulin sensitivity. Rosiglitazone can be used alone or in combination with metformin. A low incidence of side effects was noted in clinical trials. If you have heart failure, fluid retention, or active liver disease, your health-care provider will evaluate you to decide if Avandia is appropriate.

Troglitazone (Rezulin)

You may have heard of the drug *troglitazone*, brand name Rezulin, used in the past as a treatment for diabetes. An insulin-sensitizing agent, the drug improved glucose tolerance and insulin resistance and was commonly prescribed for women with PCOS. However, in March 2000, it was taken off the U.S. market by the FDA. Rezulin was associated with potentially serious side effects, including a few cases of liver failure and death.

Because of the problems with Rezulin, physicians are more likely to monitor liver function when prescribing similar medications such as Glucophage, Pioglitazone, and Rosiglitazone.

Insurance Restrictions

You may have a problem getting insurance to pay for insulin sensitizers if you don't have diabetes. Currently, the FDA has approved Glucophage, Pioglitazone, and Rosiglitazone only for type II diabetes. A drug not having FDA approval for a specific illness or condition is considered by insurance companies as an "off-label" use. It may be medically sound to take the drug, but formal approval for PCOS has not been given. FDA approval may be more forthcoming at some point; clinical studies are underway all over the world using insulin-sensitizing drugs in the treatment of PCOS. Insurance companies may be more likely to reimburse if you suffer from hyperinsulinemia (elevated blood insulin levels) or insulin resistance in connection with PCOS. Also, an insurance company may be more willing to pay if your doctor sends them a non-formulary request in which he/she explains the benefits of the medication and why it is being prescribed for PCOS.

It may be difficult to get a prescription for insulin sensitizers to treat PCOS because it is an off-label use. Physicians may not want to risk the liability. Take research with you to your doctor's office and determine if he or she is willing to research the matter.

Oral Contraceptives

Oral contraceptives are known also as the Pill, OCs, BCs, BC tablets, or birth control pills. They usually contain two types of hormones, estrogen and progestin. When taken properly, they prevent pregnancy. Oral contraceptives work by stopping a woman's egg from developing each month.

Traditionally, physicians have prescribed oral contraceptives to regulate menstrual periods in women with PCOS. Used properly, oral contraceptives can help a woman menstruate every four weeks. Because they cause women to menstruate regularly and shed the uterine lining, oral contraceptives are also one of the choices to help reduce a woman's risk of endometrial cancer. Studies have shown that using oral contraceptives decreases by 50 percent a woman's lifetime risk of developing endometrial cancer, the most common gynecological cancer.

Types of Oral Contraceptives

Oral contraceptives come in three basic types: monophasic, biphasic, and triphasic. Each type contains the hormones estrogen and progestin in varying amounts.

The progestin has an antifertility affect, suppressing ovulation. The three types differ in the amount of both hormones they produce throughout the woman's cycle.

Monophasic

A *monophasic* pill provids a level daily dose of the hormones estrogen and progestin. For 21 days you take the same strength of both hormones (one color), plus seven inactive tablets (another color) to complete your 28-day cycle. The inactive tablets are included so that women do not get out of the habit of taking a pill daily.

Biphasic

With *biphasics*, the estrogen level usually stays the same, but the progestin level is increased in the later part of the cycle. The reason for this variation is to try to more closely mimic a woman's natural cycle. If you are using a biphasic 21-day pill, you will take tablets of one strength (color) during the first part of your cycle and tablets of a second strength (color) during the second part of your cycle. The exact number of days you will take each strength varies depending on the medication, but it will always add up to 21. With a 28-day biphasic prescription, during the last seven days of your cycle you will take a third colored pill that is hormonally inactive.

Triphasic

Triphasic pills are the newest advancement in oral contraceptives and are designed to most closely mimic the natural menstrual cycle. If you are using a triphasic 21-day pill, you will take three varying doses of hormones, with each pill a different color. The number of days at each dosing level varies from 5 to 10, depending on the prescription. With a 28-day triphasic prescription, you will take an additional seven inactive tablets, which are a fourth color.

Some women respond well to birth control pills. As Missy, age 22, explained, "I am taking a combination pill, with both estrogen and progesterone (progestin). I took one for years that was just the progesterone type and it worked well, but after the birth of my twins it wasn't strong enough. I seemed to bleed and spot all month. I switched three months ago, and so far so good. I have stopped losing hair on my head, and I have stopped growing hair where I don't want it. My cycles are also right on time. I have always had good luck with birth control pills for controlling PCOS symptoms."

Yet some women have reported a worsening of PCOS symptoms while taking triphasics, also called tricyclics. The first phase has such a low estrogen dose that it may not properly suppress the growth of the cysts and the other PCOS symptoms, and it may well exacerbate the symptoms. There may be other reasons that haven't yet been fully explored.

"The first pill I was on was a tricyclic," said Shelly, 29. "It was great for four years, and then I started having 'Dr. Jekyl-Mr. Hyde' mood swings. I had a lot of stress in my life at that time, which the doctor said could have contributed to the new PMS symptoms. He switched me to a monophasic pill. The mood swings went away, but my periods were extremely heavy, requiring changes of a maximum tampon with pad backup every two hours. When I became anemic about a year later, I switched types of pills again and tolerated them well."

Choosing an Oral Contraceptive

Oral contraceptives are a good treatment option for many women. Most have few side effects. However, experiences with oral contraceptives can vary widely from woman to woman. The effects of birth control pills on our bodies is complex, and there are many individual variations on PCOS. Accordingly, there is no uniform recommendation for the right medications to manage PCOS symptoms. The best advice: Proceed with caution. If you are on an oral contraceptive, it's a good idea to monitor your condition carefully. Keep written records, and make sure your doctor is monitoring you closely, too. If you think the pills are worsening your condition, tell your doctor right away. If you have taken a pill for a couple of months and think you are reacting poorly to it, ask your physician about switching you to another type. If you were prescribed an oral contraceptive in the past and did not do well with it, let your physician know.

Side Effects of Oral Contraceptives

For most women, taking oral contraceptives does not create problems. Side effects, if any, usually occur during the first three months of use. Check with your doctor as soon as possible if any of the following side effects occur:

- Changes in the uterine bleeding pattern at menses or between menses
- Decreased bleeding at menses
- Breakthrough bleeding or spotting between periods
- Prolonged bleeding at menses

- An occasional stopping of menstrual bleeding
- A complete stopping of menstrual bleeding that occurs several months in a row

Less common side effects include headaches or migraines, increased blood pressure, and vaginal infection with vaginal itching or irritation. Women with diabetes mellitus may experience a mild increase in blood-sugar faintness, nausea, pale skin, or sweating.

Other side effects may occur but usually diminish as your body adjusts to the medication. However, check with your doctor if any of the following side effects persist:

- Abdominal cramping or bloating
- Acne (usually less common after the first three months and may improve if it already exists)
- Breast pain, tenderness, or swelling
- Dizziness
- Nausea
- Swelling of ankles and feet
- Unusual tiredness or weakness
- Vomiting
- Brown, blotchy spots on exposed skin
- Gain or loss of body or facial hair
- Increased or decreased interest in sexual intercourse
- Increased sensitivity of skin to sunlight
- Weight gain or loss

For some women with special health problems, oral contraceptives can cause more serious side effects. These can include benign (noncancerous) liver tumors, liver cancer, or blood clots or related problems, such as a stroke. The following side effects may be caused by blood clots. Get emergency help immediately if any of the following side effects occur:

- Abdominal or stomach pain (sudden, severe, or continuing)
- Coughing up blood; headache (severe or sudden)
- Loss of coordination (sudden)
- Change in or loss of vision (sudden)
- Pains in chest, groin, or leg (especially in calf of leg)
- Shortness of breath (sudden or unexplained)
- Slurring of speech (sudden)
- Swelling, weakness, numbness, or pain in arm or leg

Although these side effects are rare, they can be serious enough to cause death. Such risks are increased from smoking cigarettes. Risks also increase with age. You may want to discuss your risk of these side effects with your doctor.

Drugs for Inducing Menstruation

Many women with PCOS take medications monthly to induce their periods. However, these medications do not cause ovulation. If you wish to become pregnant, it will likely be necessary to take other medications that promote ovulation. Still, it is possible to become pregnant while using period-inducing medications if you ovulate spontaneously. The two most common medications that induce menstruation are progestins and micronixed progesterone.

Progestins

A progestin is a synthetic medication that mimics the action of the natural hormone progesterone to induce a period. The most commonly prescribed progestin is *medroxyprogesterone acetate (Provara)*. If your estrogen levels are adequate, your period should begin within one week of completing the medication. If your period does not begin, talk to your physician. Some women begin bleeding while they are in the middle of taking this medication. If this occurs, ask your doctor about stopping the medication.

Micronized Progesterone (Prometrium)

Taken orally, this drug also can help start the menstrual cycle. It is not a synthetic drug; rather, it is a natural progesterone that originates from a plant extract or, in some cases, is extracted from horse urine. It is close to your body's progesterone. Prometrium is reported to have fewer side effects than Provera, although some women cannot tolerate either.

Consider Hysterectomy Carefully

Clearly, a *hysterectomy* (removal of the uterus) is necessary in some cases, expecially if there is cancer or pre-cancerous changes of the endometrium. However, this surgery is not an appropriate medical treatment for PCOS. Unfortunately, a hysterectomy is often recommended by physicians who are not knowledgeable about current PCOS treatment options. If your physician suggests hysterectomy for PCOS, it is important to seek a second opinion and to gain a full understanding of exactly why this procedure is being suggested and why other treatment options are not appropriate in your case. Typically, a hysterectomy does not eliminate many of the PCOS-related symptoms, including the weight and unwanted hair. The bottom line is, gather as much information as possible and be an informed consumer before you make any important treatment decisions.

D-chiro-inositol

This drug is still waiting approval by the FDA; however, drug trials have been encouraging. The women who took the drug, as part of a scientific study, showed decreases in insulin and testosterone levels. And, the majority of the women in the study ovulated. The drug has not been reported to have problematic side effects. Its effects on pregnancy are unknown.

5

Getting Pregnant

All Mary ever wanted was to be a mom. Even as a little girl, she loved to rock her baby brother and sing him to sleep. She was the most sought-after baby-sitter on the block as she grew older. But now, at age 41, being around babies makes her sad. It's a painful reminder that she and her husband are still childless. Mary is not alone. Infertility strikes about one in seven couples trying to become pregnant. PCOS is one of the leading causes of infertility.

Mary had three years of treatment managed by her gynecologist, who tried repeated rounds of fertility medication but without success. It wasn't until she decided to go to a reproductive endocrinologist that she was diagnosed with PCOS. Together, they agreed she had other treatment options. Mary is still waiting but feeling more hopeful now that she has found a fertility specialist.

Infertility and PCOS

Many women with PCOS have difficulty becoming pregnant due to their irregular menstrual cycles, or lack of cycles. Irregular cycles can make it extremely difficult to pinpoint when or if ovulation is occurring. Fortunately, there are many treatments now available to promote ovulation. In addition, some women with PCOS who do occasionally ovulate can become pregnant without fertility treatments. Overall, even though some women with PCOS are unable to become pregnant, a great number of women do conceive and have successful pregnancies, either on their own or by undergoing fertility treatments.

Choosing a Fertility Specialist

One of the first steps to successfully managing your fertility treatments is finding a good physician. You want to find a fertility specialist—someone who primarily treats women and couples with fertility problems. Most likely, this will be a reproductive endocrinologist (RE). An RE is usually trained as an OB/GYN and has received additional training in reproductive endocrinology. When choosing an RE, look for one who is board certified and who has completed a two- to three-year fellowship in reproductive endocrinology, a specialty in which the physician focuses specifically on how hormones affect reproduction and pregnancy. He/she should be very knowledgeable about PCOS and be thorough, attentive, and compassionate with you and your mate.

A fertility specialist should want to talk with you extensively before beginning any treatment, to find out both your and your partner's medical history and your overall goals for achieving pregnancy. He/she should also be available to answer any questions and concerns as they come up. Furthermore, since fertility, especially ovulation, can be somewhat unpredictable, you may want to find someone with weekend and/or evening office hours so that if you experience complications or need to go in for testing, you can be seen right away.

Below are a few other questions you should consider before selecting a fertility specialist.

- **Who is recommending the specialist?** Make sure whoever is recommending the fertility specialist is reputable and qualified to make such a recommendation. If you have a good OB/GYN or family physician, he/she is most likely qualified to help you find an appropriate fertility specialist.

- **What is the specialist's background?** Ask if the fertility specialist is board-certified and how many years he/she has been working with patients having difficulty conceiving, especially those with PCOS. Also, you might want to ask your fertility specialist about his/her pregnancy rates as well as live birth and multiple birth rates.

- **Does the specialist have experience in working with women with PCOS?** Since REs are highly specialized, they are able to provide a wider range of treatments such as fertility drugs, advanced reproductive technologies, and surgical options.

- **Does the specialist have experience monitoring fertility drugs?** Once you decide to take fertility drugs, you want to be closely monitored to avoid complications and increase your chances of becoming pregnant.

- **Is the specialist qualified to do surgery?** If the fertility drugs do not work and you want to look into surgery, you want to make sure your fertility specialist is qualified to do such surgery.

- **What will treatment cost?** You want to know up front what to expect and how much money everything will cost. Fertility treatments can be expensive and may not be covered by insurance. Also, make sure your fertility specialist's office has experience in working with insurance companies to ensure that they will make every effort possible to help you negotiate with your insurance company to possibly cover costs. (Sometimes diagnostic tests such as blood work and ultrasounds are covered by insurance.)

Methods to Monitor Ovulation

The first step in achieving pregnancy is to determine whether you are ovulating. Once you know that you are ovulating, you can plan intercourse to maximize your chances of becoming pregnant. Your physician may suggest several methods to monitor your cycle to determine when ovulation is occurring.

Basal Body Temperature (BBT)

One way to determine whether you are ovulating is to check your *basal body temperature (BBT)*, your body's temperature at rest. It should be taken at the same time each day—right before you get out of bed in the morning and after at least six hours of sleep. It can be taken orally, vaginally, or rectally. Most women choose to take their temperature orally. Either a mercury or a digital thermometer can be used. However, most women choose a battery-operated digital thermometer. Although it is more expensive, a digital thermometer is safer (virtually unbreakable) and easier to read, reducing the time needed to record your temperature.

Each day, your temperature should be charted on a special piece of graph paper. (Your physician can likely give you copies.) A cycle in which ovulation has occurred is characterized by a *biphasic temperature chart*. This means your temperature remains lower until the time of ovulation, when a rise occurs of about 0.2 degrees centigrade or more. The rise takes place abruptly soon *after* the egg is released. The rise is the result of increased progesterone levels. The temperature remains at the higher level until just before, or at the onset of, the next period. If you do not see a change in temperature, you are most likely not ovulating.

Anything unusual—a cold, a late night, drinking alcohol, or any stressful situation—can affect your temperature. Therefore, many women find it difficult to chart BBT. Even a half-hour delay in taking your temperature can reduce reliability.

Note: charting BBT can only indicate whether you have *already* ovulated. Therefore, it is not useful in timing intercourse to achieve pregnancy during that cycle. By the time your temperature has gone up, it is generally too late to conceive. However, some researchers indicate there is a slight temperature drop just prior to ovulation. The information is useful for knowing when you might try intercourse during the next cycle. Still, since women with PCOS have irregular cycles with varying lengths, it can be impossible to predict when ovulation will occur the next month. Accordingly, charting BBT may be most helpful in determining whether your cycles are typically ovulatory or not. In addition, BBTs can be useful when planning to do multiple cycles of Clomid.

Examining Cervical Mucus

Another way to monitor cycles is to determine the color and consistency of cervical mucus. This may be done using either your fingers or toilet paper. In most women, cervical mucus varies from dry, to sticky, to creamy, to "egg-white" just before ovulation.

Good cervical mucus at the time of ovulation is important to fertilization since it provides an optimal environment for sperm.

During a typical 28-day cycle, the consistency of cervical mucus should be as follows:

Days 1-5	Menses
Days 6-9	Dry, or little or no mucus
Days 10-12	Sticky, thick mucus, becoming less thick and whiter
Days 13-15 (most fertile time)	"Egg-white" mucus—thin, elastic, slippery, clear
Days 16-21	Sticky, thick mucus
Days 22-28	Dry mucus

When mucus is described as dry, this means you won't find much mucus to the touch. Sticky refers to having enough mucus to feel sticky between your fingers. The mucus may be creamy and feels somewhat like lotion when you rub your fingers together. The so-called egg-white mucus resembles raw egg whites. It can be either clear or streaked and stretches an inch or more. This represents a woman's most fertile time in the cycle. Since every woman is different, changes in cervical mucus can sometimes be hard to notice.

Pain, also called *mittelschmerz*, or cramping in the ovaries right about the time of ovulation may also indicate that ovulation, or rupture of the mature follicle, is occurring. Some women can determine ovulation by checking their cervical position.

By becoming more familiar with your body, you might be able to gain better insight into how your reproductive system is working.

Ovulation Predictor Kits (OPKs)

Ovulation Predictor Kits (OPKs) are sold over the counter and use urine to detect the LH surge that occurs just *before* the egg is released from the ovary. OPKs are especially useful if you are taking fertility medication. Since OPKs let you know right before the egg is released, you can use OPKs to plan intercourse.

There are many different brands of OPKs, including many name and generic brands. OPKs generally cost about $20 to $30 for 5 days worth of tests. Most OPKs are simple to use. Urinate on the test stick, and about 5 to 10 minutes later, it will determine whether you are having an LH surge by measuring the amount of LH in your urine. Usually, there are two lines on the test stick—the test line and the control line. If the test line is a lighter shade than the control line, you are not having an LH surge. If the test line is the same or a shade darker than the control line, an LH surge has been detected. Once the LH surge has been detected, you will most likely ovulate within the next 24 hours.

To ensure you catch the LH surge, you should begin testing a few days before you think you are going to ovulate. If you are taking fertility medication, talk to your doctor about when you should start testing since fertility medication can change the length of your cycle or affect the test by causing a false positive.

Unfortunately, many women with PCOS cannot use OPKs since their LH levels might be high enough to give a false positive result. Since different OPKs measure LH at slightly different levels, you might want to try a few different brands when you are certain you are not ovulating so see if you get a false positive.

One product that might help women with PCOS determine their LH surge is a *fertility monitor*. It is similar to the traditional OPK in that it determines the LH surge by measuring the amount of LH in your urine. However, it uses actual numerical values instead of colored lines to record your LH level. This allows women with high levels of LH to still notice an LH surge by watching the numbers increase. This product costs about $200, plus the cost of replacement test sticks.

Diagnostic Tests to Monitor Ovulation

The most reliable way to determine if and when ovulation is occurring is to undergo a series of diagnostic tests performed by a physician. These tests are usually done in conjunction with charting BBT, noting cervical mucus, and/or using an OPK to determine the LH surge.

Postcoital Test

Once an LH surge is detected, you will be instructed to have intercourse and then go to the doctor's office for a postcoital test, which consists of taking a swab of your cervix (it will probably feel like a Pap test) to look at the amount and quality of the sperm present and the condition of the cervical mucus. This is important because some fertility medications, such as clomiphene citrate, can actually cause changes in the cervical mucus that inhibit conception.

Transvaginal Ultrasound

Earlier, we discussed the transvaginal ultrasound for use in diagnosing PCOS. It can also be used to determine whether a woman is ovulating. In this case, the ultrasound is usually done after the postcoital test. The ultrasound is used to actually see your ovaries and to check the uterine lining. The doctor can examine the size of your ovaries to see exactly how many follicles are developing (which lets you know if you are at risk for multiple births) and how big they are. To be considered "ripe" and the optimum size for conception, follicles should measure about 16-20 millimeters in diameter. And, the uterine lining should be about 10-12 millimeters thick to sustain a pregnancy.

7 Day Post-Ovulation Progesterone Test

At about Day 21 in your cycle (or about 7 days after you think you have ovulated), you might be asked to come in for a 21-Day progesterone test, or mid-luteal serum progesterone test. This test will tell you if your egg was released from the ovary. If it was released, your progesterone level should be significantly higher. If your progesterone levels are low, the egg most likely was not released.

Most often these tests are administered to women taking fertility medication. Some doctors suggest that women have an ultrasound, a postcoital test, and a progesterone test during each cycle. Other physicians only recommend one or two of these tests during a cycle.

Ultimately, the more closely your cycle is monitored, the better understanding you and your doctor will have about how to correct any problems.

Period or Pregnancy?

If you did indeed ovulate successfully, you should begin your period exactly 14 days after the egg was released. If you do not get your period 14 days after you ovulated, you might be pregnant. If this occurs, take a pregnancy test. If it comes back negative, wait a few days and retest. If it is still negative and you still have not started your period, call your doctor for further information. If it is determined that you did not ovulate, then your doctor may prescribe medroxyprogesterone acetate or micronized progesterone to induce your period so you can start another cycle.

If you charted your basal body temperature, your temperature will stay high if you are pregnant. If your temperature starts dropping, then your period is impending.

Common Fertility Medications

The major benefit of taking fertility medication is that you may have a greater chance of becoming pregnant. These drugs work by stimulating egg production, encouraging ovulation, or by stabilizing hormone levels which may be disrupting the fertilization process. Fortunately, a number of such medications are available for women with PCOS, but not every medication works for everyone.

In addition to the potential side effects listed with each drug, some studies indicate fertility medication, especially long-term use, may be associated with ovarian cancer. Another risk is ovarian hyperstimulation syndrome (OHSS), a rare but serious condition in which the ovaries enlarge as a result of fertility medication and cause abdominal pain or discomfort, bloating, or nausea. More severe forms of OHSS can involve blood clots, massive accumulation of fluid in the abdomen and pelvis (requiring surgical drainage), and damage to other organs such as the lungs, liver, and kidneys.

Clomiphene Citrate

Clomiphene citrate, also known by the brand names Clomid and Serophene, is usually the first fertility medication given to women with PCOS. It works by causing the body to produce more FSH and LH, the hormones that promote egg growth. Once the brain senses increased estrogen levels, it signals the LH surge that results in ovulation.

While it may take several months to determine the right dosage of clomiphene citrate, the drug should not be taken for an extended period of time, even if it causes you to ovulate. It can actually have a negative effect on fertility by causing thick cervical mucus, which is hostile to sperm and inhibits fertilization. Additionally, taking the drug for longer than six months is unlikely to result in a pregnancy. If your doctor continues to recommend this treatment, it is reasonable to seek another opinion. Clomiphene citrate is fairly inexpensive, costing about $25 for five 50-milligram pills.

If a woman is going to ovulate on clomiphene citrate, she usually does so in the first three or four cycles. Some studies estimate that about 75 percent of women will ovulate on clomiphene citrate, with about 35 percent achieving pregnancy.

Unfortunately, many women with PCOS are "Clomid resistant." This means that they do not ovulate with clomiphene citrate, even at the maximum dosage. Recent studies have shown that clomiphene citrate, when taken with an insulin sensitizer such as metformin, significantly increases ovulation and the chance of pregnancy.

There are several potential side effects of clomiphene citrate, including breast tenderness, headaches, depression, and fatigue. There is also an increased risk of conceiving twins or triplets. However, other potential side effects can be more serious. It's possible to experience ovarian enlargement, even ovarian hyperstimulation. Other, rare side effects that need to be reported immediately to your physician include changes in vision and severe headaches. It is best to stop the medication immediately if you develop these symptoms.

Gonadotropins

Gonadotropins are drugs that stimulate the ovaries to produce and release eggs. The medications act by supplying a woman's body an extra amount of the hormones FSH and LH, or FSH only—the hormones that start egg production. The risks with gonadotropins include an increased chance of multiple births and ovarian hyperstimulation. The risk of multiple pregnancy is around 20 percent, with most of these being twins. The chance of ovarian hyperstimulation is less than 1 percent per cycle if managed by competent doctors. Other possible side effects vary greatly from one woman to the next but may include bloating, abdominal pain, nausea, insomnia, hot flashes, and depression. The most common gonadotropins are listed below.

FSH

Because women with PCOS have an elevated LH level, sometimes pure FSH is given to balance out the LH to FSH ratio. Once there are adequate levels of estrogen and the follicle develops, an hCG shot is given to release the egg.

There are different types of FSH available, depending on how it is prepared. Common types of FSH that are prescribed include Fertinex, Gonal-F, and Follistim. FSH is given by daily injection and is usually expensive. Side effects include mood swings and ovarian hyperstimulation.

Human Menopausal Gonadotropin (hMG)

More popularly known as Pergonal, Humegon, and Repronex, this medication is an extract from the urine of menopausal women and contains LH and FSH, which stimulate ovulation. hMG is given by injection, usually in the thigh or buttocks. A shot of hCG is then given later in the cycle to promote the release of the egg. Some research suggests that about 90 percent of women ovulate using HmG but only about 60 percent actually conceive.

hMG is expensive, costing more than $1,000 per cycle, and the risk of multiple births can be as high as 20 percent. Mood swings can be a side effect. Also, nearly 20 percent of women who take hMG may develop ovarian hyperstimulation if not monitored properly.

Human Chorionic Gonadotropin (hCG)

The drug hCG is used with other fertility medications, including clomiphene citrate, FSH, and HmG, to promote ovulation by triggering the LH surge. In some women with PCOS, a follicle successfully develops during the use of other fertility medications, but the egg is never released. By performing a transvaginal ultrasound about the time ovulation should occur, the doctor can view the developing follicle. If the follicle appears "ripe" but the LH fails to trigger the release of the egg, the doctor can give an injection of hCG. This should cause ovulation.

Insulin Sensitizers

Increasingly, insulin sensitizers such as Avandia and metformin are considered the most effective methods for treating infertility in women with PCOS since they bring insulin levels into balance. Many women with PCOS who did not previously ovulate while taking ovulation induction medications alone (including women who were Clomid resistant) successfully ovulated while using insulin sensitizers. By using insulin sensitizers in conjunction with clomiphene citrate or another fertility medication, over half of women with PCOS will ovulate.

Some physicians will prescribe insulin sensitizers only if your insulin or glucose test confirms that you have insulin resistance. However, using insulin sensitizers to treat infertility has proved helpful for many women without such indications, such as those who have "normal" or "borderline" glucose levels and are not yet insulin resistant. Talk to your physician to find out if taking insulin sensitizers as part of your fertility treatment is right for you.

Ovarian Surgery

Ovarian surgery is another option for women wishing to become pregnant. Surgery is not a cure for PCOS, but it can be performed to promote ovulation long enough to become pregnant. Most physicians recommend ovarian surgery only after medications have failed. There are two types of ovarian surgery—ovarian drilling and wedge resection.

Of these two methods, *ovarian drilling* is the most common. It is an outpatient, laparoscopic procedure that uses a laser to pierce the thickened coat of the ovary. The surgeon uses the laser to penetrate the cysts on each ovary. Fluid is drained from the ovary, eliminating many of the cysts. In turn, the amount of androgens produced is lowered, causing a decrease in LH.

About 80 percent of women undergoing this procedure will ovulate and about 30 to 40 percent will become pregnant. Women at or close to ideal body weight usually have better results after surgery than those that are overweight. Risks involved with ovarian drilling include the normal risks of surgery, such as bleeding and infection. Although it is a noninvasive procedure, ovarian drilling still carries the risks of possible adhesions and excessive destruction of the ovary, which could result in ovarian failure.

Wedge resection, a major procedure in which cysts are surgically removed from the ovaries, was used successfully in the management of women with PCOS prior to the availability of antiestrogens in the 1960s. It resulted in a high rate of ovulation but was followed by significant formation of adhesions that prevented pregnancy a few months after the procedure was performed. The procedure is seldom used today.

Advanced Reproductive Technologies

Some women with PCOS who are not successful at getting pregnant using traditional methods of treating PCOS-related infertility turn to advanced reproductive technologies (ARTs). These procedures are carried out daily in the more than 300 fertility clinics across the nation. These procedures can be extremely expensive and can carry many risks, including multiple births and high rates of miscarriage.

The success rates of ARTs are quite variable. Success depends on many factors, including: age, other medical or reproductive problems (both male and female), the experience of the medical team and clinic, the quality of the eggs and sperm, the number of embryos implanted, and the number of cycles attempted, to name just a few.

Some studies have shown that PCOS women tend to produce many eggs, but have lower fertilization rates than other woment undergoing IVF. Consequently, if you are interested in finding out more about ARTs, you should consult a reproductive endocrinologist or other fertility specialist for an individual evaluation. He/she can assess your specific medical situation and your chances of success using ARTs.

Intrauterine Insemination (IUI)

For this procedure, egg production is stimulated through the use of fertility medications and monitored closely by the attending physician. As soon as it is clear that the woman is successfully ovulating, sperm from her partner or donor is deposited directly into the uterus. This commonly done when hostile mucous is present. The intent is to concentrate the number of healthy, moving sperm, shortening the distance to the ovary by bypassing the vagina, cervix, and most of uterus, and accurately timing the meeting of sperm and egg shortly after ovulation. The cost of the procedure averages $200-$300 per cycle.

In Vitro Fertilization (IVF)

In vitro fertilization (IVF) involves retrieving the eggs from a woman's ovaries and and fertilizing them with sperm in a laboratory. Once fertilization occurs, the fertilized egg or eggs are returned to the uterus for implantation. The cost ranges from between $8,000 to $20,000 per cycle.

Gamete Intrafallopian Transfer (GIFT)

In this procedure, eggs are first taken from the ovary. Then sperm and eggs are simultaneously placed directly in the *fallopian tubes,* the tube through which the egg travels from the ovary to the uterus. The physician is guided by a laparoscope, a narrow probe, containing an optic scope, which allows him/her to see the internal organs. This procedure is used much less frequently than in vitro fertilization. Costs for GIFT can range from $11,000 to $15,000 per cycle.

Zygote Int   *Transfer (ZIFT)*

ZIFT i   ~ the ovary, which are
then fertili   embryos are
placed in'   : cost of this
procedur

Intracyt

In   1 into an egg
through   lting embryo is
transfer   edure is about
$10,50

Dono

                                    another woman.
The   n from a mate or
don   nside the uterus.
Alth   she will carry the
bab   runs from $12,000
to

O

                                    n get pregnant and
su   ll women with PCOS
ca   heir not being able to

conceive, and advanced reproductive technology does not work for all women. After months and sometimes years of treatment, the medical costs and emotional price tags can be high. As such, many couples are faced with making difficult choices. They may decide to remain child-free or choose to bring a child into their family through surrogacy, adoption, or foster care.

Maintaining a Pregnancy

Several researchers have indicated that the risk of miscarriage in patients with PCOS may be slightly higher, with the miscarriage rate being between 39 and 54 percent. However, studies of couples seeking pregnancy have shown that as many as 50 percent of all pregnancies are lost, with the majority of them being lost early and not clinically recognized. Infertile couples appear to have a slightly higher miscarriage rate than fertile couples. Many factors can contribute to miscarriages both for women with PCOS and those without, including:

- Age (After age 35, as age increases, so do miscarriage rates.)
- Fertility treatments (Advanced reproductive technologies carry a greater chance of miscarriage.)
- History of recurrent miscarriages
- Genetic defects
- Other fertility problems, such as uterine abnormalities
- Hormonal imbalances

The more risk factors you have the higher your risk of a miscarriage. Many endocrinologists now believe that pregnancy in women with PCOS carries elevated risks of miscarriage, diabetes, and other problems. Accordingly, it is important to see your health-care provider as soon as possible after you discover that you are pregnant.

Some health-care providers may want to wait until you are eight weeks pregnant before they see you. If you have PCOS, it is recommended that you not wait this long. The sooner you see your health-care provider, the sooner he/she can help you maintain a healthy pregnancy by starting to monitor you.

However, most pregnant women with PCOS can see a regular OB/GYN or midwife for their prenatal care. Some women, especially those with diabetes or hypertension, may be referred to an OB/GYN who specializes in high-risk care. The health-care provider may use any of several methods to help maintain your pregnancy.

Supplementing Progesterone

Women with PCOS are often prescribed progesterone supplements if their progesterone levels are too low to sustain a pregnancy. During the first trimester of pregnancy, the mother's body produces the hormone progesterone to keep the uterus in good condition to support the pregnancy. After the first trimester, the placenta takes over producing the progesterone.

If a woman is not producing enough progesterone during the early part of pregnancy, a miscarriage will occur. Fortunately, if the progesterone level is checked early on and a low level is noticed, she can take progesterone supplements during the first 12 weeks of pregnancy. This will help raise her progesterone level enough to sustain the pregnancy until the placenta can take over.

Insulin Sensitizers to Prevent Miscarriage

According to one preliminary, small study, the insulin sensitizer metformin, taken throughout pregnancy, reduces first-trimester miscarriage from 45 to 9 percent in women with PCOS. Another study indicates it isn't safe to stop taking metformin when pregnancy is achieved. Many of the original forty-three women in the study conceived on metformin. This raised the difficult question of whether to continue the medication throughout the pregnancy. Initially, as soon as pregnancy was confirmed, the metformin was stopped. But researchers were stunned by an ensuing first-trimester miscarriage rate greater than 50 percent as well as by the frequent (about 30 percent) development of pregnancy- induced hypertension.

Despite early indications that women can safely take metformin during pregnancy, it is still controversial. There are no reports of birth defects in children whose mothers take metformin throughout pregnancy. However, there have not been any long-term studies of difficulties for the mothers or children.

Other Fertility Problems

Sometimes women with PCOS can also have other fertility problems such as endometriosis, fallopian tube blockage, uterine abnormalities, and excess prolactin (the hormone that stimulates milk production). Or, perhaps male factors such as inadequate sperm may be a problem. It is important before any fertility treatments are started to rule out other fertility problems that might complicate the situation. This may include a semen analysis or having a *hysterosalpingogram* (*HSG*), in which dye is injected into the uterus and fallopian tubes and X-rays are taken to look for abnormalities or blockages.

Still, other times there may be no apparent reason for a woman's infertility. This can occur when everything seems to be working—the cycle is normal, ovulating is occurring, the eggs are of good quality, the amount of sperm is adequate, and the cervical mucus is good. But still there is no pregnancy. If this happens to you, talk to your physician about what to do next. Your physician may order more extensive testing or recommend a break from fertility treatments to give your body and your mind a well-deserved rest.

Secondary infertility can strike both couples with and without PCOS. While it is not true in all cases, some women with PCOS who had little or no difficulty conceiving their first child end up having tremendous difficulty getting pregnant a second time. This could be due to several factors, including increased age, continued changes in hormone levels, increased weight gain, or worsening of PCOS.

Pregnancy-Related Concerns

Much more research is needed in this area. According to surveys, anecdotal evidence, and some physicians, women with PCOS face a greater risk of complications during pregnancy. In particular, gestational diabetes, and preeclampsia (toxemia) and eclampsia are frequently cited in women with PCOS.

Gestational Diabetes

Women with PCOS may be more likely to develop gestational diabetes, or glucose intolerance, during pregnancy. Gestational diabetes is usually discovered during the 24th to 28th weeks of pregnancy with routine screening. The symptoms are usually mild and not life-threatening to a pregnant woman; however, the increased maternal fasting glucose levels are associated with an increased rate of fetal or newborn deaths. Maintaining control of blood glucose levels significantly reduces the risk to the offspring. The infant born to a woman with gestational diabetes may have an increased birth weight, low blood glucose levels during the early newborn period, and be jaundiced. The risk factors for gestational diabetes are a maternal age over 25 years, a family history of diabetes, obesity, a birth weight over 9 pounds in a previous infant, the unexplained death of a previous infant or newborn, a congenital malformation in a previous child, and recurrent infections.

Symptoms of Gestational Diabetes:

- Increased thirst
- Increased urination
- Weight loss in spite of increased appetite
- Fatigue
- Nausea
- Vomiting
- Infections (including bladder, vaginal, skin)
- Blurred vision

The goals of treatment are to maintain blood glucose levels within normal limits for the duration of the pregnancy and to ensure the well-being of the fetus. Fetal monitoring to assess fetal size and well-being may include ultrasound exams. Diet management provides adequate calories, nutrients, and control of blood glucose levels. Nutritional counseling by a registered dietician is recommended. Exercise can also be very effective in controlling gestational diabetes.

If dietary management does not control blood glucose levels within the recommended range, your doctor may consider insulin therapy. Blood glucose self-monitoring is required for effective treatment with insulin.

High blood glucose levels often resolve after pregnancy. However, women with gestational diabetes should be followed postpartum and at regular intervals for early detection of diabetes. Up to 30 to 40 percent of women with gestational diabetes develop overt diabetes mellitus within 5 to 10 years after delivery. The risk may be higher if the woman is considered obese. Many doctors recommend increasing the number of glucose tolerance tests for pregnant PCOS patients. Exercise and avoiding sugary beverages are thought to be helpful.

Preeclampsia and Eclampsia

There are some indications that women with PCOS may be more likely to develop preeclampsia, also known as pregnancy-induced hypertension or high blood pressure. If left untreated, preeclampsia (also called toxemia) can develop into eclampsia, a full-blown form of the illness. Eclampsia is a serious problem, and is the leading cause of maternal death. However, if proper medical care is given, it is very unusual for eclampsia to develop.

Symptoms of preeclampsia include:

- Edema (swelling of the hands and face, or severe swelling anywhere on the body)
- Weight gain (unintentional) in excess of 2 pounds per week (Gain may be sudden over 1 to 2 days.)
- Headaches that don't go away with treatment
- Decreased urine output
- Nausea and vomiting

- High blood pressure or elevated blood pressure
- Agitation
- Chest or upper abdominal pain
- Proteinuria (protein in urine)
- Thrombocytopenia (a decrease in the number of circulating blood platelets)

The exact cause of preeclampsia has not been identified. Numerous theories about the causes exist, including genetic, low-protein intake, vascular (blood vessel) and neurological factors. None of the theories have yet been proven. Preeclampsia occurs in approximately 5 percent of all pregnancies. Increased risk is associated with first pregnancies, teenage mothers, mothers more than 40 years old, African-American women, multiple pregnancies, and women with a history of diabetes, hypertension, or kidney disease. Because many women with PCOS are insulin resistant, obese, and may have hypertension, the risks are greater.

Although there are currently no known prevention methods, it is important for all pregnant women to obtain early and ongoing prenatal care. This allows for the early recognition and treatment of conditions such as preeclampsia. "I developed preeclampsia three and a half weeks before my due date. I had slowly started having problems and one day my blood pressure shot through the roof. My daughter was born later that night. It was incredibly frightening," Anna, 23, remembered. The best treatment for preeclampsia is bed rest and delivery as soon as possible for the baby. Patients are usually hospitalized, but occasionally they may be managed on an outpatient basis with careful monitoring of blood pressure, urine checks for protein, and weight. Optimally, the condition may be managed until a delivery after 36 weeks of pregnancy can be achieved.

In severe cases of preeclampsia with the pregnancy beyond 28 weeks, delivery is the treatment of choice. For pregnancies less than 24 weeks, the induction of labor is recommended, although the likelihood of a viable fetus is minimal. Prolonging such pregnancies has shown to result in maternal complications as well as infant death in approximately 87 percent of cases. Pregnancies between 24 and 28 weeks present a "gray zone," and conservative management may be attempted, with monitoring for maternal and fetal complications. Because there are not clear guidelines for less severe cases of preeclampsia, frequent follow-up of fetus and mother is necessary, as is continued revision of the treatment plan with changes.

Maternal deaths caused by preeclampsia are rare in the United States. Fetal or perinatal deaths do sometimes occur, yet the chance of death decreases as the fetus matures. The risk of recurrent preeclampsia in subsequent pregnancies is approximately 33 percent. Preeclampsia does not appear to lead to chronic high blood pressure.

Macrosomia

Women with PCOS, who are overweight or who have gestational diabetes, may have large fetuses. This condition is known as macrosomia. This can sometimes result in difficult births and Cesarean sections.

Breast-feeding

Currently, there is little research to determine whether PCOS affects breast-feeding. Many women with PCOS are successful when it comes to breast-feeding; others experience the same difficulties as women in the general population. Some research indicates there may be problems with milk supply. Pregnant women who wish to breast-feed should find a lactation consultant prior to delivery in case one is needed.

6

Alternative Treatments

K im, age 20, didn't like taking every new drug that came down the pike. She wasn't opposed to medical treatments, she just wasn't sure she wanted to try medications that hadn't been around for longer than a couple of years. She didn't want to be a "guinea pig," and she preferred natural methods of healing. As she gathered information, Kim realized that she had to begin from scratch to create her own treatment plan for the symptoms of PCOS.

Kim spoke with her physician and made an appointment with a naturopath. Her doctor admitted that he didn't know much about natural treatments, but he was willing to be helpful if he could. He did insist on regular monitoring of her insulin levels to see if her insulin resistance worsened and suggested that she have at least four periods a year. Treatment goals in hand, Kim wanted to try natural treatments.

Alternative Therapies

Some women with PCOS, especially those who do not wish to take hormones, find relief from symptoms through alternative therapies such as herbs, acupuncture, homeopathic remedies, and other alternative approaches. It is very important, however, to discuss your choices with your health-care professional, in addition to seeing a naturopath.

Naturopaths typically recommend an assortment of approaches in an attempt to harness the body's natural healing ability to boost the immune system, restore good health, and prevent disease. The whole person is considered—emotional, genetic, and environmental influences included. Tenets of naturopathy also include a diet high in fruits, vegetables, and whole grains. Noninvasive physical therapy techniques may offer relief from a variety of muscle and joint complaints. Treatment may include any of the following, depending on your symptoms and the practitioner's experience and philosophy:

Homeopathic Remedies: Homeopathy is a medical practice based on the principle that diseases can be cured by drugs that produce the same effects as the symptoms of the disease. Such drugs essentially work in the same way as vaccines do in preventing infection and illness. Homeopathic remedies are diluted solutions of assorted herbs, animal products, and chemicals.

Dietary Restrictions: Vegetarianism or the elimination of certain food categories (such as dairy products) is recommended to relieve sensitivity reactions and clear the body of toxins. Dietary advice often includes instruction on "proper combining" of groups.

Physical Medicine: Manipulation of the muscles, bones, and spine, and physiotherapy using water, heat, cold, ultrasound, and exercise, are used to relieve a broad array of ailments.

Stress Reduction: Counseling, hypnotherapy, biofeedback, and other methods are used to heal physical damage from stress.

Detoxifying Regimens: Fasting, using enemas, and drinking large amounts of water help purify the body.

More of a philosophical approach to health care than a particular form of therapy, naturopathy endeavors to cure disease by harnessing the body's natural healing powers. It takes very seriously the medical motto "first, do no harm." The success of naturopathy varies greatly depending on individuals and conditions. Mainstream doctors are also gaining new respect for certain antioxidant vitamins as potential agents against disease, and some are even acknowledging the effectiveness of certain herbs.

A number of women with PCOS experiment with natural treatments for their symptoms. Note: many women have achieved regular menstrual cycles with these treatments but have *not* ovulated. Subsequently, they still are infertile. Additionally, natural treatments may not work well for insulin resistance. It is also important to note that natural treatment for women with PCOS is not based on scientific research. Most of the evidence is anecdotal and a specific natural treatment has not been established.

Potential for Side Effects

"Natural" does not always mean "safe." The greatest hazard is that using naturopathic therapies without any conventional advice could allow a serious medical condition to go undiagnosed and unchecked. There is little or no scientific proof that many time-honored tools in the naturopathic toolbox do what they are purported to do. The naturopathic notion that illness arises from vaguely defined "toxins" in the body that must be purged through fasting, enemas, sweating, and water consumption has not been verified through clinical research. Some herbal preparations can be quite toxic, and excessive fasting or use of enemas can upset the body's balance of fluids and minerals, leading to potentially dangerous consequences such as irregular heartbeat.

Accordingly, drastic dietary restrictions can undermine good health and should generally be avoided, especially by the very young, the elderly, and those with a medical condition (such as diabetes) that requires special dietary modifications. Likewise, many popular food supplements, as well as the mega-dose use of vitamins, have so far failed to show definitive effects. In fact, a few have even proved harmful. Naturopathic use of "natural" hormone preparations are also questionable, since the potency of these products can vary to dangerous degrees.

Also, you should always exercise caution if you are pregnant, trying to become pregnant, or breast-feeding. If a dietary recommendation seems extreme, your wisest course is to first seek the approval of a registered dietician or a conventional physician knowledgeable about nutrition.

Choosing a Therapist

Naturopathic remedies are offered by a variety of other health-care providers, including chiropractors, nutritionists, holistic nurses, and massage therapists. However, if you want the complete package, you need to seek out a *doctor of naturopathic medicine* (*ND*). Such practitioners have completed four years of graduate-level training at a naturopathic medical college. If your practitioner has a high level of medical expertise, diagnosis may also involve laboratory analysis, allergy testing, X-rays, and a physical exam.

In the states where they are currently licensed, naturopathic physicians ust pass either a national or state-level board examination. Their scope of allowable practice varies from state to state. Some states grant certification in specialties such as natural childbirth or acupuncture.

Although naturopathic physicians have considerable medical training, they are not necessarily qualified to diagnose and treat urgent or potentially life-threatening conditions. Responsible naturopathic physicians refer such cases to more appropriate medical specialists. If you have symptoms that may indicate PCOS, consult a regular physician first, then a naturopathic practitioner if you desire.

Herbal Therapies

In recent years, the use of herbal therapies has increased. Despite this increased use, it is important to understand the Food and Drug Administration does not regulate herbal therapies. Accordingly, herbal preparations have not undergone the same kind of rigorous testing that prescription drugs go through before being made available to the public. As a result, there are no purity standards for herbals, and there is no proof that the herbs actually do what they are claimed to do. Herbs should be used with caution and guidance.

"I have used herbal treatments, based only on my thorough research. I was not under the care of a holistic practitioner," explained Leslie, a woman with PCOS. "However, I made sure I found out which herbs could be toxic and should be used only under the care of a practitioner. That's the one thing that makes me nervous—so many people think all herbs are safe, and that's not the case. It is not safe to begin self-prescribing a handful of herbs that sound good."

Additionally, herbs may have additional ingredients which may or may not be listed. For example, California health officials recently investigated several companies' natural Chinese herbs after diabetic herb users had several episodes of hypoglycemia, and discovered the products also contain the prescription diabetes drugs *glyburide* and *phenformin*. California's health department concluded that herb users are at risk if they also take regular diabetes medicine. The FDA has stopped imports of the products.

The herbals listed below are those used with varying degrees of success by some women with PCOS. It is very important to note that the herbs listed here are not regulated by the FDA, and in most cases, there is no scientific data to back up claims about their effectiveness. And in fact, because herbs may contain powerful substances, they have the potential to cause harmful interactions with other drugs. Again, self-medicating with these herbs is not recommended. Consider using herbal remedies only with the help of a trained professional.

Chaste tree berry (Vitex agnus-castus)

This herb is thought to increase production of the luteinizing hormone (*LH*) and prolactin. Some consider it useful to stimulate milk flow and to regulate the menstrual cycle when there is excessive bleeding, too frequent, or prolonged menstruation. Women who have PMS with significant depression should probably avoid chaste tree berry. Some research suggests that PMS with depression is caused by excess progesterone, and chaste tree berry is said to raise progesterone levels. Those with high LH levels should likely avoid this herb as well.

Black cohosh (Cimicifuga racemosa)

Like chaste tree berry, black cohosh is said to enhance the pituitary secretion of luteinizing hormone with subsequent ovarian stimulation. It contains isoflavone constituents, which are believed to bind to estrogen receptors in the body.

Blue cohosh (Caulophyllum thalictroides)

This herb is purported to be a uterine tonic, suggesting it may relax a hypersensitive uterus as well as increase the muscular tone of a weak uterus.

Saw Palmetto

Saw palmetto is a palm that grows throughout the southeastern United States. The herb's active ingredient is unknown, but studies in Europe show that an extract from the berries appears to counteract the effects of androgens. As an anti-androgen substance, it may be effective in treating excessive hair growth in women. There are two forms of saw palmetto, the berries and the extract.

Cinnamon

From ½ to ¾ teaspoon of cinnamon with every meal is said to help keep insulin and blood sugar levels under control. It contains a phytochemical called methyl hydroxy chalcone polymer (MHCP) which improves cellular glucose utilization and increases the sensitivity of insulin receptors.

Damiana

Damiana is thought to be a remedy for impotence, but its effectiveness is largely unconfirmed. In homeopathic medicine, it is used for female sexual disorders. It is thought to stimulate muscular contractions of the intestinal area and bring oxygen to the genital area. It also may inhibit iron absorption rates.

Dong quia (Angelica sinensis)

Used for menstrual irregularities and infertility, dong quai is purported to tone a weak uterus by promoting metabolism within the organ, regulating hormonal control and improving the rhythm of the menstrual cycle. However, if you are trying to conceive, there is some indication that it may cause birth defects.

Glutamine

Glutamine is an amino acid which has been shown in animal studies to prevent high blood pressure and high insulin levels in mice that were susceptible to developing high sugar levels when fed a high-fat diet. Polyunsaturated fatty acids (omega-3 and omega-6 fatty acids) help keep cell membranes flexible. Flexible cell membranes have more and better insulin receptors, which improves glucose metabolism.

Garcinia cambogia

An extract from Garcinia cambogia is thought to help tune up the body's glucose and insulin metabolism. The garcinia fruit, native to India and southeast Asia, is a rich, natural source of hydroxy-citric acid, or HCA. HCA works to block a key cellular pathway that converts glucose into fat. Animals fed an HCA-supplemented diet have shown reduced food intake, a decline in body fat and lowered triglyceride levels.

Licorice (Glycyrrhiza glabra)

This plant contains hormonally active compounds categorized as saponins. A Japanese study found licorice-based medicines improved menstruation in women with infrequent periods. The study also found that licorice helped women with elevated testosterone and low estrogen levels, as commonly occurs in polycystic ovary disease.

Milk thistle

Milk thistle is said to help the liver and it is often used to cleanse the system. Some naturopaths recommend milk thistle to anyone who is taking any kind of medication to help keep liver enzymes normal, even if the liver enzymes are already normal.

Motherwort (Leonurus cardiaca)

This herb is said to affect the nervous, cardiac, and female reproductive systems. It is used by some individuals for anxiety, tension, nervous disorders, menopause, premenstrual syndrome, and other hormonal imbalances. Motherwort is also considered by some to be a uterine tonic, useful for cramps as well as uterine weakness.

Progesterone creams

Some women report success with using a progesterone cream to produce regular periods by helping to restore proper hormone balance. Natural progesterone, given before ovulation, can inhibit the levels of LH and in effect block ovulation as both ovaries "think" the other one has released an egg.

The natural progesterone creams get mixed reviews from clinicians, and not many support using them. On the other hand, some physicians prefer transdermal (absorbed through the skin) natural progesterone in cream or oil formulation; the cream is absorbed more efficiently and the effect lasts longer, without the emotional highs and lows from oral drugs. The cream may be applied to the palms, face, neck, upper chest, breast, inside of the arms, or behind the knees.

The key criterion is the amount of progesterone (in milli-grams) contained in a given natural progesterone product. Under healthy conditions, a premenopausal woman's system produces about 20 mg daily of progesterone between days 15 and 26 of the cycle. While amounts in the range of 20-30 mg daily are often sufficient, relief from the primary symptoms will indicate a woman is taking the appropriate dosage.

If you have been using progesterone cream and think you might be pregnant, be sure that you aren't expecting before you stop using it because it is possible that suddenly stopping could cause a miscarriage. Some women use wild yam cream instead, thinking it is a natural alternative. However, it is not the same and does not have the same benefits.

Siberian Ginseng (Eleutherococcus senticosus)

This and other tonic botanicals is purported to improve fertility by enhancing overall health and vitality. Siberian ginseng is also said to act on the brain to promote regulation of repro-ductive hormones.

Squaw vine (Mitchella repens)

Used by Native Americans as a fertility and pregnancy tonic, squaw vine is a uterine tonic that is reported to increase uterine circulation and reduces uterine congestion. Some claim the herb also improves uterine tone and relaxes uterine spasm.

Tulsi

Tulsi, or sacred basil (Ocimum sanctum), is an herb from India. The leaves are chewed with the intent of helping the body process starchy and sugary foods. Tulsi has been used in traditional Indian remedies to help control high blood glucose levels for more than 700 years.

Unicorn root (Chamalerium luteum)

A uterine tonic, unicorn root, also called blazing star, is said to be useful for women who have a tendency toward pelvic congestion, a condition typically experienced as a sensation of heaviness. This herb may help prevent miscarriage and menstrual bleeding due to uterine weakness. This is often found in women's herbal compounds.

Wild yam (Dioscorea villosa)

Wild yam contains plant hormones including the steroidal saponins diosgenin, pregnenolone, and botogenin. In its crude form, wild yam has a weak hormonal activity in the body that may help prevent habitual miscarriage due to hormonal insufficiency. The creams sold as "wild yam" are not the same as progesterone cream. Although wild yams are used in the manufacturing of progesterone, they do not have the same effect or measurable effects as the standardized formulas.

Acupuncture

Some women believe that acupuncture can help restore ovarian function. Acupuncture involves the stimulation of certain points on the skin by the insertion of needles. The procedure has been used as a treatment in Asia for several thousand years but has not been proven effective by modern medical standards. While some studies have suggested that acupuncture improves ovulation, more studies need to be completed to determine its effectiveness on women with PCOS.

The World Health Organization has listed forty conditions for which claims of the effectiveness of acupuncture have been made. They include acute and chronic pain, rheumatoid and osteoarthritis, muscle and nerve "difficulties," depression, smoking, eating disorders, drug "behavior problems," migraines, acne, ulcers, cancer, constipation, and more.

The frequency of complications of acupuncture is not known, since no survey has been done. Nevertheless, according to medical journals, serious complications occur even in experienced hands. These include fainting, local hematoma (bleeding from a punctured blood vessel), pneumothorax (punctured lung), convulsions, local infections, hepatitis B (from unsterile needles), bacterial endocarditis (an infection that can affect women with mitral valve prolapse), contact dermatitis, and nerve damage. There is also the risk that a lay acupuncturist will fail to diagnose a dangerous condition.

Reflexology

Is the foot a microcosm of the entire body? Reflexologists say it's true. They press on various "reflex points" along the foot to relieve symptoms elsewhere in the body. Although they don't promise to cure the underlying cause, they do believe that their technique can alleviate a wide variety of stress-related problems, as well as headaches (both tension and migraine), premenstrual syndrome, asthma, digestive disorders, skin conditions such as acne and eczema, irritable bowel syndrome, and chronic pain from conditions such as arthritis and sciatica. Some people suggest that reflexology can help alleviate many symptoms associated with PCOS.

Finally, with so many alternative therapies available, it may be difficult to choose one that will help you. The bottom line is, the natural methods may work for a while for some people, and for some specific symptoms, but they do not work for everyone and may not address the root cause of the problem.

7

Long-Term Risks of PCOS

Susan, 40, had experienced PCOS-related symptoms for as long as she could remember. In fact, when she was in her mid-20s, her doctor suspected that she had PCOS and told her so. Susan really hadn't thought about it since. Even though the symptoms could sometimes be annoying, they never really bothered her too much. Susan was a successful businesswoman, sometimes working fourteen hours a day and almost always working on the weekends. Susan had just gotten married, bought a new house, and was now in the middle of making major renovations. Susan and her new husband had decided that they did not want to have children. Both wanted to remain career focused. Taking care of their cat was about all the responsibility that they wanted to handle.

As a result, Susan really wasn't concerned about her irregular periods. She actually thought of herself as lucky, not having to worry about it every single month. As she was looking through the newspaper one Sunday afternoon, she noticed an article about PCOS in the health section. The article mentioned something about new research that linked PCOS to heart disease and diabetes. Susan was surprised to read this and wondered if she should see a doctor about her PCOS.

Insulin Resistance and Diabetes

Diabetes mellitus is a serious disease in which the body cannot process insulin properly. In the United States alone, 15.7 million people have diabetes. It is the seventh leading cause of death. There are two main types of diabetes: *type I* (also called *juvenile* or *insulin-dependent diabetes*), which usually begins during childhood or adolescence, and *type II* (also called *adult-onset* or *non-insulin-dependent diabetes*). Type II is the most common form of diabetes, making up 90 to 95 percent of all diabetes cases that occur in adults.

It is estimated that at least half of all women with PCOS have detectable insulin resistance. All women with PCOS who have insulin resistance are at serious risk for developing type II diabetes at some point in their lives. In fact, everyone who develops type II diabetes most likely has insulin resistance first. The problems caused by insulin resistance just get worse until the body is no longer able to utilize the insulin at all. This results in diabetes.

Unfortunately, there are often few or no symptoms at all to alert you that this is happening. Women with PCOS should have their blood tested regularly for insulin resistance and diabetes. You are at even higher risk for developing type II diabetes if you:

- Weigh 20 percent more than your ideal body weight
- Have high blood pressure
- Have low HDL cholesterol levels (under 35 mg/dl)
- Have high triglyceride levels (over 200 mg/dl)
- Have a close relative with diabetes

- Are from a high-risk ethnic group
- Are over age 40
- Have delivered a baby weighing over 9 pounds
- Have a history of gestational diabetes

Type II diabetes is a chronic condition that has no cure. In people with type II diabetes, glucose (a form of sugar) builds up in the blood. However, with proper treatment, your blood sugar levels can return to normal again. A "normal" sugar level does not mean you are cured and no longer have diabetes. Instead, it shows that your treatment plan is effective, that you are doing a good job of controlling your diabetes.

The goal for treating diabetes is to lower your blood sugar (glucose levels) and improve your body's use of insulin. This can be achieved in a variety of ways, including meal planning, exercise, weight loss, and taking medications.

Since your body breaks down food into glucose, your blood sugar level rises when you eat. You want to exercise good meal planning that slows down this rise in sugar. You want to try to choose foods that are low in fat, have protein, and contain only moderate amounts of carbohydrates. Many nutritionists and dieticians specialize in helping people who either have diabetes or who are at risk for developing diabetes make better meal choices in order to successfully manage their blood sugar levels.

Being active also helps your body to more efficiently process glucose and utilize insulin. If you don't currently exercise, you might want to become more active. Ideally, you should be active on most days of the week for a total of 30 minutes per day, which can be broken down into shorter five to ten minute sessions. If you are not used to exercising regularly, start slow. Even a

5-minute walk is good. However, before you start any exercise plan, you should always talk to your health-care provider first.

Losing weight is another big part of managing diabetes. It will help you utilize insulin better. Ask your health-care provider how much weight you should lose. Also find out the most effective way for you to lose weight. Sometimes, just losing 10 or 20 pounds is enough to better control your diabetes.

Physicians often prescribe insulin sensitizers to help control diabetes and bring glucose and insulin levels back to "normal." However, taking these medications does not replace the need for healthful habits, including eating well and exercising.

If not successfully managed, diabetes can lead to serious medical complications including heart disease, stroke, eye and kidney problems, and problems involving the blood vessels, nerves, and feet. It is important to mention that these treatment methods for controlling type II diabetes can also be effective in managing insulin resistance. Women with PCOS who maintain appropriate blood glucose and insulin levels can significantly lessen the risk of developing diabetes while also minimizing some of the other effects of PCOS.

Cardiovascular Disease

Researchers are beginning to understand the connection between PCOS, heart disease, and stroke. In the past few years, numerous studies have found that women with PCOS have a seven times greater risk of developing cardiovascular disease than women without PCOS. This is probably due to the fact that women with PCOS also tend to have more of the risk factors associated with cardiovascular disease.

The major risk factors for heart disease and stroke are:

- Cigarette/tobacco smoking
- High blood cholesterol (over 200)
- High blood pressure (over 120/80)
- Physical inactivity
- Heredity (family history of cardiovascular disease, especially if early onset)
- Male gender
- Other contributing factors such as increasing age, diabetes, obesity, and stress

Unfortunately, PCOS often results in many of these risk factors. Women with PCOS have a greater tendency to be overweight or obese. PCOS can also cause a woman to develop high blood cholesterol levels and even an increase in blood pressure. The risk for heart disease increases for women with PCOS who smoke, have a family history of cardiovascular disease, are under a lot of stress, or are physically inactive. The bottom line is, the more risk factors you have, the greater chance you will develop cardiovascular disease, which could result in a heart attack or stroke.

To lower your risk for heart disease and stroke, it is important to seek treatment. By directly treating PCOS, one might be able to bring hormone levels into a normal range, minimizing or eliminating the symptoms and effects of PCOS, including high cholesterol and insulin levels. In some cases, there may be a need for additional medications such as those for high cholesterol and high blood pressure.

Also, it is important to make appropriate lifestyle changes as part of your treatment plan to prevent heart disease. Being overweight and physically inactive can significantly increase your chance of developing heart disease. Talk to your physician about safe and effective ways to lose weight and increase your exercise. It is important that any weight loss plan you choose takes into consideration your PCOS.

Endometrial Hyperplasia

Since most women with PCOS do not have normal menstrual cycles, the uterine lining is not shed and replaced each month. As a result, old cells continue to build up within the uterus. The more time that passes without a period, the more buildup that occurs. Sometimes this buildup can cause *endometrial hyperplasia*, an overgrowth of the endometrium, which can be a precursor to cancer. There are several degrees of hyperplasia. *Simple hyperplasia* holds the least risk for developing endometrial cancer, whereas hyperplasia with *atypia* (a pathological term for the presence of abnormal, precancerous cells) holds a much higher risk—50 percent or greater.

The longer you go without a period, the greater your chance of developing endometrial hyperplasia and perhaps cancer. This is why it is important to seek medical help if you have abnormal or absent periods. Many women with PCOS think that if they are not trying to become pregnant it is okay to miss periods. Most physicians do not advise women to go more than a few months without a period.

Cancer

If left untreated, endometrial hyperplasia can develop into cancer of the uterus or the endometrium. If your physician is concerned that your uterine lining is too thick, placing you at risk for developing endometrial or uterine cancer, he/she might suggest that you have a *dilation and curettage* (D&C), in which the cervix is opened and the lining of the uterus is surgically scraped out. After the procedure is completed, most women experience bleeding and abdominal cramping for a few days. Your physician may also order an *endometrial biopsy* so that a portion of the endometrial tissue can be examined in the lab. Both D&Cs and endometrial biopsies are outpatient procedures done under local anesthesia.

Women with a family history of cancer or increased levels of estrogen face an even greater risk of developing endometrial cancer. The primary way to reduce your risk for developing endometrial or uterine cancer is to make sure that you see your health-care provider for a complete gynecological exam each year. He/she can help you maintain regular periods, which should also reduce your risk. For example, he or she may prescribe birth control pills which have been shown to reduce the risk of endometrial cancer by more than 50 percent. The effects of insulin sensitizing agents on endometrial cancer risks are unknown.

8

The Emotional Impact

"I spend so much of my day thinking *Why Me?* Why do any of us have PCOS? Why is this our curse in life? Did we get shown a choice, and this was the one we picked?" asked Nan, a 36-year-old woman with POCS.

"I have a hard time believing that. I just don't get it. No matter how many hours I wrack my mind and soul, I do not understand. And that is the biggest of all the wounds inflicted on me—that this is the mindless bad luck of the genetic draw. That I can't fix it. That it will never get better. That it is destroying my heart and soul bit by bit, day by day. How do I hang on? How do I manage?"

Depression

PCOS can be frightening, overwhelming, and discouraging. Fear about health issues, grief about a loss of control over family planning, and anger at years of misdiagnosis are all common reactions. When you add the side effects of multiple medications, it can seem hopeless. Women can suffer depression as a side effect of PCOS, or they may feel depressed because of

PCOS-related difficulties. It can be difficult to know which came first, the depression or the PCOS. Depression can manifest itself in physical symptoms such as:

- Headaches
- Stomach problems
- Insomnia
- Loss or sudden increase of appetite
- Sudden change in menstruation

Emotional symptoms may include:

- Emptiness
- Sadness
- Hopelessness
- Guilt
- Remorse

Cognitive or behavioral changes may also occur, including:

- Loss of concentration
- Memory loss
- Lack of libido
- Inability to respond sexually
- Withdrawal from social interactions

Some women with PCOS remember being depressed even in childhood. "I can look at myself in pictures from an early age and see an enormous sadness, even at age 4," said Nina, a 35-year-old with PCOS. "By my early 20s, I felt as though I was going insane. My body was so out of whack and it was crying out for help. I always felt as though there was a black cloud over me."

Depression and Infertility

Infertility and subfertility are difficult emotional hurdles. PCOS robs a woman of many things, cruelest of all her ability to conceive naturally and build a family. Many women first learn that they have PCOS because they have sought the help of a fertility specialist. By that time, they typically have been trying to get pregnant for a year or more. Infertility alone is a particularly trying experience, but combined with PCOS, it can be traumatic. "It's an emotional one-two punch," according to Kristin Rencher, executive director of PCOSA, the Polycystic Ovarian Syndrome Association, "knowing that your infertility is a permanent condition that can't be solved by surgery or simple fertility awareness methods. Discovering that you are at elevated risk for life-threatening medical conditions is also frightening. The good news is, the more we learn about PCOS, the more tools we have to restore fertility and to avoid heart disease, cancer, and diabetes."

Treating Depression

Depression can be treated a number of ways. Often, talk therapy with a professional counselor can help. Some individuals may benefit from counseling in a group setting, where they feel less isolated and benefit from the experiences of others.

Prescription antidepressants are also frequently used to treat clinical depression and may be an appropriate choice. There are no specific antidepressants used for patients with PCOS. However, women may have to switch types before they find the one that works best for them.

"I have had to the accept the fact that my hormonal changes wreak havoc with my moods and well-being, if I don't intervene with an antidepressant," said Susan, 36.

"I am simply not willing to feel depressed. I take a low-dose antidepressant and am grateful to have my 'real' personality back. I'm more positive, creative, and focused, and a lot less worried."

Nevertheless, women are sometimes afraid of being diagnosed as depressed. They may not want it in their medical records, or they are concerned that needing an antidepressant is somehow a weakness. "The stigmas about depression/anxiety and medication are finally shifting away in our society. I look forward to the day when, like diabetics and heart disease patients, depression can be treated openly without shame. Depression can require medications just like other illnesses," said Nancy.

Embarrassment

Side effects like acne, hirsutism, and obesity can cause women to feel less than feminine and bring up issues about self-worth. Our culture somehow expects women to be thin, to have flawless skin and smooth, hairless bodies. Women with PCOS may not look like that ideal and may feel ashamed of the way they look. Embarrassment from physical symptoms as well as the difficulty of living with infertility can leave women feeling isolated and withdrawn. Some women are reluctant for partners to see them nude, because of their weight.

Stress and Anxiety

Stress is defined as a feeling of tension that is both emotional and physical. Women with PCOS may experience stress about infertility treatment, health-care choices or expenses, or the reality of living with a chronic illness. Different people perceive different situations as stressful. Stress management is intended to help reduce tension. It involves making emotional and physical changes. The degree of stress and the desire to make the changes will determine the level of change required.

One's attitude plays an important role. It can influence whether a situation is stressful. A person with a negative attitude will often perceive many situations as stressful. Negative attitude is a predictor of stress.

Physical well-being is an important part of controlling our moods. If our nutrition is poor, our bodies are stressed and we are not able to respond well to stressful situations. As a result, we can be more susceptible to infections. Poor nutrition can be related to unhealthy food choices, inadequate food intake, or an erratic eating schedule. A nutritionally unbalanced eating pattern also means an inadequate intake of nutrients. Inadequate physical activity can further result in a stressful state for the body. A consistent program of physical activity can contribute to a sense of well-being.

"I can't say this enough—even simple walking is a good stress releaser. Add it to your routine. Not only will it help increase your utilization of excess insulin and androgens, it will also help you deal with stress and will help relieve depression, too!" said Rebecca, 32.

Tips for Stress Relief

- Refocus negative thoughts to be positive.
- Talk positively to yourself.
- Plan some fun.

- Make an effort to stop negative thoughts.

Physical activity:

- Start an individualized program of physical activity.
- Decide on a specific time, type, frequency, and level of physical activity.

Nutrition:

- Plan to eat foods for improved health and well-being.
- Eat an appropriate amount of food on a reasonable schedule.

Social support:

- Make an effort to interact socially with people.
- Reach out to individuals.
- Nurture yourself and others.

Relaxation:

- Use relaxation techniques (guided imagery, listening to music, prayer, etc.). Learn about and try different techniques, then choose one or two that works for you.
- Take time for personal interests and hobbies.
- Listen to your body.
- Take a mini-retreat.

If you're unable to manage stress, consider the help of a licensed social worker or psychotherapist who can help. Scheduling time with one of these professionals is often helpful in learning stress management strategies and relaxation techniques.

Finding Support

There aren't any easy answers. We need people in our lives who cherish us, support us, and encourage us. If we do not currently have such people, then we need to actively seek them out. They might be in your church, place of employment, family, etc. If you are trying to conceive, your reproductive specialist will often have a professional counselor who can meet with you and/or offer support groups such as RESOLVE.

Professional Support

Professional support is provided by both medical practitioners and mental health experts. The first line of defense is a good doctor who not only diagnoses your problem but treats you with understanding and works with you to find the right solution to your problems. However, for many women this alone is not enough; they benefit from sharing their feelings and experiences with other women who are dealing with the same problems.

Peer Support

Peer support is provided by the Polycystic Ovarian Syndrome Association (PCOSA), an international support and education organization for women with PCOS. The organization has several different avenues for peer support, including local chapters and Internet forums. Many who participate in the chapters and forums find this to be one of the best forms of therapy. Sharing with others can lighten the load. Person-to-person support is provided through the network of local chapters.

Every day PCOSA receives hundreds of e-mails. Information is exchanged. Lists are available for those women who want children, those who are not trying to conceive, teens, women in menopause, and even general PCOS support. To subscribe to an online e-mail support group, you can log on the PCOSA web page and enroll at www.pcosupport.org. You can choose to have each e-mail delivered as it arrives, or in digest form, as one complete package daily. Bulletin boards do not involve e-mail but allow you to post or respond to topics regarding PCOS. Like the mailing lists, they offer discussions of a number of different topics.

"Up until very recently, women with PCOS have tended to suffer in silence. Now we communicate often," explained Kristin Rencher. "It's challenging enough to get up the nerve to tell your doctor that you have excess hair growing on your chin or breasts, let alone mention it to your husband or friends. The emotional support from others who have PCOS is invaluable. Peer support offers the ability to talk freely about the issues you have been dealing with. It can be especially wonderful to talk with others who have firsthand knowledge of what you are going through."

Friends and Family

It is usually a relief to finally know that the odd constellation of symptoms you experience are attributable to one medically recognized disorder. The next problem is, do you share that information with your partner, family, and/or friends? If so, how? It is especially important that you help those who live with you understand PCOS and what it is doing to your body. Once they understand how PCOS affects you, they can be active participants in your healing. Your partner may be able to shed insight or help you identify patterns.

Families and friends can support women by learning more about PCOS, attending PCOS support group meetings, encouraging healthy choices, and simply asking what they can do to help.

9

Hope for the Future

Since childhood, Brianna, 36, had always been interested in the medical field. She earned a degree in nursing and loved working as a nurse in a busy pediatrician's office. Because of her medical background, Brianna immediately wanted to know what research was being conducted to learn more about PCOS. Fortunately, her doctor taught classes at the local medical school, so he put her in touch with a researcher who was conducting a study about diet and PCOS.

Brianna signed up for the study right away. It was a simple research study that only lasted a few months. She was asked to keep a log of everything she ate and to answer a number of questions about her nutrition, exercise habits, and her PCOS symptoms. Brianna really felt good about being part of a study that might help other women with PCOS. Now she volunteers occasionally at the medical school, educating other women about participating in studies.

Research Studies and Clinical Trials

An extraordinary amount of research is currently being done to find out more about PCOS. Women with PCOS have the opportunity to be involved in this cutting-edge research by participating in research studies and clinical trials.

A basic *research study* gathers and interprets information. It usually involves participants answering questions via a survey or interview.

A *clinical trial* is a well-planned research study that involves the administration of a test treatment, such as a drug. In most cases, those who receive treatment are compared to a *control group* that does not receive the treatment. Any differences between these two groups are noted and perhaps studied further.

To make the studies more effective, clinical trials are often masked, or blinded. That is, some information is withheld from either the study participant and/or the physician conducting the study. Clinical trials can be single-blind, double-blind, or triple-blind. In *single-blind trials*, usually the study physician knows whether the study participant is assigned to the treatment or control group, but this information is not given to the participant. In *double-blind trials*, neither the study physician nor the study participant knows to which group the participant has been assigned.

Finally, in *triple-blind trials*, no one, not even the researchers responsible for the trial, knows to which group each participant belongs. These are rare with medication trials since a monitoring committee will ordinarily review the data periodically to ensure there is no harm to the participants. Once the trial is completed, all the information is released. However, it may be months (even years for some larger trials) before the information is available to local investigators and participants.

Participation in a Clinical Trial

If you are interested in participating in a research study or clinical trial, first ask your physician about any research that is being conducted in your area. You can also contact your local medical school or teaching hospital (usually a hospital that is affiliated with a medical school or university). Most often, it is the endocrinology or gynecology departments that are interested in conducting research on PCOS. In addition, you can also find out about national studies by contacting the National Institutes of Health in Bethesda, Maryland. PCOSA keeps an up-to-date list of current research opportunities on its web site. Sometimes a study requires that you live close to the research center. This is especially true of clinical trials. However, some research studies are just trying to gather information and will interview women nationwide. They will simply have you complete a survey or a telephone interview.

Before participating in a clinical trial, however, you should ask the following questions:

- **Who is responsible for conducting the clinical trial?** Make sure both the researcher and the study site are reputable and have a good history of conducting clinical trials.

- **What are the participant requirements?** Many studies are specific in which types of people they need. For instance, they might be looking for women age 18 to 25 who are not interested in becoming pregnant over the next few months. Make sure you fit the requirements.

- **What commitment must be made?** Sometimes participating in a clinical trial means many trips to the study site, while others only require a single visit. Make sure you can fulfill the commitment you make. Also, make sure you know about such things as blood work, examinations, and interviews.

- **What is the compensation?** Most clinical trials offer payment or some type of compensation. Usually, the more time-intensive a trial is, the greater the compensation. Also, all associated medications, lab tests, and physical examinations should be provided at no cost to you.

- **Is the trial masked?** Will you be told whether you have been assigned to the treatment group or control group? If medication is involved, the control group is usually given a placebo so that they will not know what medication they are taking. Most likely, you will not know to which group you have been assigned until after the study is completed.

- **What is the purpose of the clinical trial?** What is this clinical trial trying to accomplish? For example, is it to study the effectiveness of a new medication? To try new methods to treat PCOS-related infertility? To determine how certain foods affect PCOS? To determine whether PCOS runs in families? Make sure you are comfortable with the goals of the trial.

- **Will you be asked to sign a consent form?** You should *always* be asked to sign a consent form before you participate in a clinical trial. This form should explain all the details of the clinical trial and tell you exactly what you should expect. You should be given the opportunity to have all your questions about the trial answered. If you have any unanswered questions or are unclear about any aspect of the study, do not sign the consent form until you get the information that you need.

- **Will I learn the results of the study?** It is important to know what is going to happen after the clinical trial is completed. Will you find out if you were a part of the treatment or control group? Will you be given the opportunity to receive the treatment if it is found to be effective? Where will the results be published? How will study participants hear about the results?

Research on PCOS

Research studies and clinical trials addressing PCOS are being conducted in almost every state and in many other countries worldwide. Some of the major areas now being studied are:

- Further information about the connection between PCOS and insulin resistance
- PCOS and genetics
- New medications to treat hirsutism
- Experimental medications to manage PCOS-related symptoms
- Medications and treatments that aid in fertility for women with PCOS
- The influence of PCOS on the risk of developing heart disease
- How PCOS affects moods
- The impact of diet and exercise on PCOS
- PCOS and adolescents

Unfortunately, there is still a lot we don't know about PCOS. The good news is, we are learning more and more each day. As a result, there are already many more treatment options available for women than there were 20, 10, or even 5 years ago. As time goes by and more research is conducted, there is a good chance that PCOS will be even better controlled and perhaps one day even cured.

Resources

Organizations

Polycystic Ovarian Syndrome Association (PCOSA)

P.O. Box 80517
Portland, OR 97280
(877) 775-PCOS
www.pcosupport.org
PCOSA, also known as PCOSupport, seeks to promote awareness of PCOS and to serve as a support system with accurate information for women with this syndrome. Membership is open, but primarily includes women who either have been diagnosed with or believe they might be diagnosed with PCOS. Membership also includes physicians and other health-care practitioners who take interest in the evaluation and treatment of PCOS. The overall purpose of PCOSA is to promote research, understanding, and communication of the most up-to-date information concerning PCOS among its membership body.

PCOTeen

www.pcosupport.org/pcoteen/about.html
PCOTeen is a division of PCOSA. PCOTeen's goal is to let teens know that they are not alone in their fight against PCOS and its effects on a young woman's body.

American Society for Reproductive Medicine (ASRM)
(Formerly the American Fertility Society)
1209 Montgomery Highway
Birmingham, AL 35216-2809
(205) 978-5000
ASRM is devoted to advancing knowledge and expertise
in reproductive medicine and biology. ASRM provides patients with
fact sheets and FAQs (frequently asked questions) on topics related
to reproductive health.

International Council of Infertility Information Dissemination (INCIID)
P.O. Box 91363
Tucson, AZ 91363
(520) 544-9548
www.inciid.org
INCIID (pronounced "inside") is a nonprofit organization committed
to using the Internet to provide the most current information
regarding the diagnosis, treatment, and prevention of infertility and
pregnancy loss. INCIID's purpose is entirely educational, providing
patients with physician directories, fact sheets, and information about
current research in reproductive health.

RESOLVE
The National Infertility Association Since 1974
1310 Broadway
Somerville MA 02144
(617) 623-0744
www.resolve.org
RESOLVE has provided help to thousands of people experiencing
the crisis of infertility. RESOLVE's mission is to provide timely,
compassionate support and information to individuals who are
experiencing infertility issues through advocacy and public
information. RESOLVE offers a comprehensive set of services for
members, including a quarterly newsletter, a hotline for physician
referrals and specific support, publications addressing infertility,
support groups, and an advocacy network to keep you abreast of
legislative and insurance changes.

Fertility Research Foundation
1430 Second Avenue
New York, NY 10021
(212) 744-5500

American Fertility Society (AFS)
2140 11th Avenue South, Suite 200
Birmingham, AL 35205-2800
(205) 933-8494

American Cancer Society (ACS)
1955 Clifton Road
Atlanta, GA 30329
1-800-ACS-2345
www.cancer.org
ACS provides information about all types of cancer.

Cancer Information Service
National Cancer Institute
Building 41, Room 10A24
9000 Rockville Pike
Bethesda, MD 20892
800-4-CANCER
www.nci.nih.gov
The Cancer Information Service provides information about the
prevention, diagnosis and treatment of cancer.

National Diabetes Information Clearinghouse (NDIC)
1 Information Way
Bethesda, MD 20892-3560
(301) 654-3810
NDIC provides educational information about diabetes.

American Diabetes Association

1701 North Beauregard Street
Alexandria, VA 22311
www.diabetes.org
The American Diabetes Association is a resource center for diabetes information.

American Heart Association

7272 Greenville Avenue
Dallas, TX 75231
(214) 762-6300
The American Heart Association provides information about cardiovascular disease, including heart disease and stroke.

American Association of Naturopathic Physicians

601 Valley Street, Suite 105
Seattle, WA 98109
(206) 298-0125
www.naturopathic.org
This organization provides a referral directory and information about naturopathic medicine.

National Center for Complementary and Alternative Medicine

NCCAM Clearinghouse
P.O. Box 8218
Silver Spring, Maryland 20907-8218
Toll Free: 1-888-644-6226
TTY/TDY: 1-888-644-6226
FAX: 301-495-4957

American Hair Loss Council (AHLC)

401 North Michigan Avenue
Chicago, IL 60611
www.ahlc.org.
AHLC is a nonprofit organization that provides non-biased information from all viable treatment areas to individuals with hair loss. You can search for both clinical dermatologists and non-clinical members of the AHLC who provide services to people with hair loss.

American Academy of Dermatology

P.O. Box 4014
Schaumburg, IL 60168-4014
Tel: (847) 330-0230 or 888-462-DERM (3376)
Fax: (847) 330-1090
www.aad.org
AAD includes a searchable database of current members.

American Electrology Association (AEA)

Teresa E. Petricca, CPE, Executive Director
106 Oak Ridge Rd.
Trumbull, CT 06611
www.electrology.com
AEA promotes the highest standards in electrology education, practice, and ethics and champions state licensing and regulation of the profession to protect the public interest. They also offer practitioner referrals.

Society of Clinical and Medical Electrologists (SCME)

651 A1A Beach Boulevard, Suite A
St. Augustine Beach, FL 32084
(904) 460-9292
SCME is a nonprofit association of professional electrologists who strive for recognition of the practice of electrolysis.

American Council for Headache Information (ACHE)

19 Mantua Road
Mt. Royal, NJ 08061
(856) 423-0258
A nonprofit patient/health-care professional partnership, ACHE is dedicated to advancing the treatment and management of headaches and to help sufferers gain more control over all aspects of their lives—medical, social, and economic. ACHE offers a quarterly newsletter and support groups.

National Foundation for Depressive Illness
P.O. Box 2257
New York, NY 10016
(212) 268-4260
The National Foundation for Depressive Illness offers referrals to specialists in mood disorders as well as an extensive bibliography of books and information on depression.

American College of Obstetricians and Gynecologists (ACOG)
409 12th Street S.W.
P.O. Box 96920
Washington, D.C. 20090-6920
(202) 638-5577
www.acog.org
ACOG is a professional membership organization for physicians specializing in obstetrics and gynecology. ACOG also provides patients with physician directories and general patient education information about issues related to women's health.

National Women's Health Resource Center (NWHRC)
120 Albany Street
Suite 820
New Brunswick, NJ 08901
(877) 98 NWHRC or (877) 986-9742
www.healthywoman.org
NWHRC is a national clearinghouse for information and resources about women's health. Their primary goal is to educate health-care consumers and empower them to make intelligent decisions by providing patients with easy-to-understand and easy-to-reach information and services. NWHRC offers many resources (including fact sheets and question-and-answer sheets) and Internet links addressing women's health issues.

CenterWatch, Inc.

22 Thomson Place, 36T1
Boston, MA 02210-1212
(617) 856-5900
www.Centerwatch.com
CenterWatch has a wealth of information related to clinical trials, including a listing of more than 41,000 industry- and government-sponsored clinical trials as well as new drug therapies recently approved by the FDA. It is a resource both for research professionals and patients interested in participating in clinical trials.

Recommended Reading

The Carbohydrate Addict's Diet: The Lifelong Solution to Yo-Yo Dieting. Drs. Rachael Heller and Richard Heller, New American Library, 1993

Dr. Atkins' New Diet Revolution. Robert C. Atkins, M.D., Avon Books, 1998

Dr. Susan Love's Hormone Book. Susan B. Love, M.D., Random House, 1998

The Encyclopedia of Natural Medicine. Michael Murray, N.D., and Joseph Pizzorno, N.D., Prima Publications, 1991

The Fertility Sourcebook. M. Sara Rosenthal, Lowell House, 1995

Handbook of Medicinal Herbs. J. A. Duke, CRC Press, 1985

In Pursuit of Fertility: A Fertility Expert Tells You How to Get Pregnant. Robert R. Frankin, M.D. and Dorothy Kay Brockman, Owl Books, 1995

Our Bodies, Ourselves for the New Century: A Book by and for Women. Boston Women's Health Book Collective, Touchtone Books, 1998

Prescription for Nutritional Healing: An A-Z Reference to Using Drug-Free Remedies. James A. Balch, M.D., Avery Publishing, 1997

What to Expect When You're Expecting. Arlene Eisenberg, Heidi Murkoff, and Sandee Hathaway, Workman Publishing, 1996

Recommended Reading

Women's Bodies, Women's Wisdom. Christine Northrup, M.D., Bantam Books, 1998

Women's Moods: What Every Woman Should Know About Hormones, the Brain and Emotional Health. Deborah Sichel, M.D. and Jeanne Watson Driscoll, M.S., R.N., C.S., William Morrow and Co., 1999

The Zone: A Dietary Road Map to Lose Weight Permanently: Reset Your Genetic Code: Prevent Disease: Achieve Maximum Physical Performance. Dr. Barry Sears, HarperCollins, 1995

Glossary

Acne: Inflammatory disease that affects the sebaceous glands of the skin.

Alopecia: Hair loss or baldness.

Amenorrhea: Absence of menstrual periods.

Androgens: Male hormones responsible for secondary male characteristics, including hair growth, voice change, and muscle development.

Anovulation: Absence of ovulation, or monthly release of an egg, from the ovary.

Antiandrogen: Blocks the effects of androgens, normally by blocking the receptor sites, but may also inhibit enzymes that make anthrogen.

Basal Body Temperature (BBT): Temperature of the body taken at rest. Theoretically, BBT rises after ovulation has occurred.

Biopsy: Removal of a sample of tissue for diagnostic examination.

Blood sugar: Level of glucose present in the bloodstream, used by the brain and muscles as energy.

Carbohydrate: Basic component of food, composed of chains of sugars. Short chains are referred to as simple carbohydrates and include table sugar, honey, maple syrup, and fruit sugars. These simple sugars are converted by the body into glucose, which affects insulin levels. Long chains are called complex carbohydrates and include those found in starchy foods such as breads, cereals, potatoes, fruits, and vegetables. These are broken down by the body into glucose more slowly and are either used for immediate energy or are stored by the body for later use.

Cervix: Lowermost part of the uterus.

Cervical mucus: Lubricant secreted by the cervix and vaginal walls. Cervical mucus usually changes consistency around the time of ovulation to encourage fertilization.

Cholesterol: Waxy substance found in animal fat. In excess, it may contribute to narrowing the artery walls, reducing blood flow.

Clomiphene citrate: Drug most commonly used to induce ovulation. Popular brand name is Clomid.

Corpus luteum: Yellow-colored mass in the ovary formed when the ovarian follicle has matured and released its egg. Responsible for secreting estrogen and progesterone. If fertilization occurs, the corpus luteum sustains the pregnancy until the placenta is formed and takes over.

Cyst: Abnormal sac usually containing fluid or solid material.

DHEAS: An androgen secreted by the adrenal gland.

Diabetes: Disease that affects blood sugar and causes inappropriate levels of insulin. Type I, or juvenile diabetes, causes a decreased production of insulin. Type II, or adult-onset diabetes, results from resistance to insulin.

Dilation and curettage (D&C): Dilating the cervix and scraping out the endometrium (lining) of the uterus.

Dysmenorrhea: Very painful menstruation.

Ectopic pregnancy: Pregnancy that occurs when the fertilized egg implants outside the uterus, usually in the fallopian tube.

Endocrine: Pertaining to the system of the body that produces hormones.

Endocrinologist: Physician who specializes in the diagnosis and treatment of diseases affecting the endocrine system.

Endometrium: Lining of the uterus.

Endometrium hyperplasia: Overgrowth of uterine lining (endometrium), usually due to the influence of prolonged estrogen exposure.

Estradiol: Most active, naturally occurring estrogen, a female hormone.

Estrogen: Female sex hormone produced by the ovary and adrenal gland that causes the development of the female characteristics and also plays a role in menstruation and pregnancy.

Fallopian tubes: Structures located between the uterus and ovaries that are responsible for transporting the egg.

Fertilization: Joining of the sperm and egg, the first step in forming an embryo.

Follicle: cyst-like structures within the ovary that contain the immature egg.

Follicle-stimulating hormone (FSH): Secreted by the pituitary gland, this hormone causes the maturation and release of an egg each month.

Galactorrhea: Milk production and release from the breasts unrelated to nursing.

Gamete intro fallopian transfer (GIFT): Surgical procedure by which sperm and egg are injected directly into a woman's fallopian tubes.

Glucose: Simple sugar molecule, the principal sugar that circulates in the bloodstream.

Gonadotropin: Substance having a stimulating effect on the ovaries or testes.

Gonadotropin-releasing hormones (GnRH): Substances released from the hypothalamus, the part of the brain that controls reproduction, to stimulate the pituitary to produce gonadotropins, which in turn stimulate the ovary to produce sex steroids.

High blood pressure: Condition in which the heart pumps blood through the circulatory system at a pressure greater than normal. Normal blood pressure is usually below 140/90 mm/Hg. Also called hypertension.

Hirsutism: Excessive hair growth.

Human chorionic gonadotropin (hCG): Substance derived from the urine of pregnant women. This is what home pregnancy tests detect to confirm pregnancy. Stimulates the corpus luetem of pregnancy to make progesterone.

Human menopausal gonadotropin (HmG): An extract from the urine of menopausal women that contains LH and FSH. Used to stimulate ovulation.

Hyperandrogenism: Condition in which a woman has high levels of male sex hormones (androgens).

Hyperprolactinemia: Excess production of prolactin, the hormone responsible for promoting milk production.

Hypothalamus: Part of the brain responsible for maintaining body temperature, sleep, hunger, and reproduction. Controls the hormones that regulate menstruation.

Hysterosalpingogram: Diagnostic test during which dye is injected into the uterus and fallopian tubes. X-rays are then taken to determine if there are any abnormalities or blockages.

Ideal body weight: Weight goal of an individual. It takes into consideration body type, muscle mass, and bone structure.

Insulin: Hormone produced by the pancreas. Insulin converts glucose from the bloodstream into glycogen, which is stored in muscle tissue and the liver.

Insulin resistance: Failure of the body to respond properly to the insulin produced by the pancreas. Related to diabetes.

Insulin sensitizers: Group of medications originally used to treat type II diabetes but now sometimes used to alleviate many PCOS-related symptoms by helping to correct insulin resistance.

Intrauterine insemination (IUI): When a very thin flexible catheter is threaded through the cervix and washed sperm is injected into the uterus.

In vitro fertilization (IVF): Uniting the sperm and egg outside the body under laboratory conditions. The fertilized egg is then returned to the woman's body in the hope that it will implant.

Laparoscope: Fiber-optic scope inserted through the navel to view the reproductive organs.

Luteinizing hormone (LH): Hormone that facilitates the conversion of the follicle into the corpus luteum.

Menarche: Very first occurrence of menstruation.

Menopause: When menstruation has stopped for at least one year, usually around age 45 to 50. Once this occurs, a woman is no longer able to become pregnant.

Menses: Approximately monthly discharge of the unfertilized egg and the uterine lining as blood flows through the vagina.

Menstruation: Monthly cycle of hormone production and ovarian activities that prepares the body for pregnancy. If pregnancy does not occur, the uterine lining is shed, causing menses.

Miscarriage: Loss of a fetus.

Obesity: Abnormal excess of fat, usually defined as more than 20 percent over ideal body weight.

Oligomenorrhea: Light and infrequent menstrual flow.

Ovaries: Two robin's egg-sized organs that produce the egg and female sex hormones.

Ovarian cyst: Noncancerous, fluid-filled sac located in or on the ovary that usually is a normal component of the ovulatory cycle.

Ovarian hyperstimulation: Rare complication that develops when the ovaries are overstimulated during the use of fertility medications such as clomiphene citrate or HmG. The ovaries enlarge and produce more follicles. This causes a buildup of fluid in the body, resulting in sudden weight gain, abdominal pain, nausea, and vomiting.

Pituitary gland: Small gland within the brain that is responsible for regulating hormones associated with milk production and the menstrual cycle.

Placenta: Organ that develops within the uterus during pregnancy. It provides the fetus with nourishment, permits the elimination of waste products, and produces hormones needed to sustain pregnancy.

Progesterone: Hormone produced by the corpus luteum in the ovary, the adrenal gland, and the placenta (in pregnant women). It prepares the uterus for pregnancy and sustains the pregnancy.

Progestin: Name used for certain synthetic or natural progesterone agents. Usually contained in many types of birth control pills.

Prolactin: Hormone responsible for milk production.

Prostaglandins: Hormone-like substances released by the uterine lining that cause uterine contractions, resulting in menstruation.

Proteins: Compounds that contain amino acids. Found in all living matter, proteins are essential for the growth and repair of animal tissue.

Provera: Progestin medication prescribed to induce a period.

Puberty: Stage of human development between childhood and adulthood when secondary sex characteristics first become evident.

Steroids: Group of chemicals (considered hormones), many of which occur naturally in the body. Steroids can greatly affect bodily functions.

Testosterone: Male sex hormone responsible for the development of male characteristics.

Uterus: Organ in the pelvic region where the fertilized egg and fetus develops. Also called the womb.

Index

About the Authors

Angela Boss is a freelance writer, Hoosier, mom, and pastor. She is Health Education Director of PCOSA, the international PCOS support group. She also serves as Director of Communications for the local Indiana PCOS chapter. Her frequent articles on PCOS and infertility can be seen at www.suite101.com and www.conceivingconcepts. com.

Ms. Boss has a bachelor's degree from Virginia Wesleyan College, Norfolk, Virginia, and a master's degree in counseling and ministry from Virginia Union University, Richmond, Virginia. Ms. Boss is also the author of two other books, *Surviving Your First Year As a Pastor: What Seminary Didn't Teach You* (Judson Press 1999) and *Heart of a Shepherd: Meditations for New Pastors* (Judson Press 2000).

Evelina Weidman Sterling is a certified health education specialist and consultant to various nonprofit and government agencies in the area of evaluation and health services research. She previously worked for the American Association for Health Education, Health Resources and Services Administration, Gallaudet University, and the American Heart Association.

Ms. Weidman Sterling holds a bachelor of science degree in biology from Mary Washington College and a master's degree in health sciences from the Johns Hopkins University School of Hygiene and Public Health. She lives in Atlanta, Georgia with her husband and children.

Richard S. Legro, M.D., received his medical degree from the Mount Sinai School of Medicine in New York City in 1987. He completed his residency in obstetrics and gynecology at Magee Women's Hospital at the University of Pittsburgh and completed a fellowship in reproductive endocrinology and infertility at the University of Southern California in Los Angeles. Since 1993, he has been a faculty member in the Department of Obstetrics and Gynecology at Penn State University College of Medicine in Hershey, Pennsylvania.

Dr. Legro's research and clinical practice are focused on polycystic ovary syndrome—diagnosis, treatment, and genetic/environmental causes. He has published over seventy-five articles related to PCOS in medical journals and books. His research has been funded by a number of pharmaceutical companies, charitable foundations, and the National Institutes of Health. He has spoken about PCOS throughout the world and has received numerous awards for his research on the syndrome. He and his family reside in Hershey, Pennsylvania.

Addicus Books Consumer Health Titles

Please send:

_____ copies of _____
(Title of book)

at $ _____each   TOTAL: _____

Nebr. residents add 5% sales tax   _____

Shipping/Handling
   $4.00 for first book.
   $1.10 for each additional book   _____

TOTAL ENCLOSED: _____

Name_____

Address_____

City _____State _____Zip_____

❑ Visa ❑ MasterCard ❑ American Express

Credit card number_____Expiration date _____

Order by credit card, personal check or money order. Send to:
Addicus Books
Mail Order Dept.
P.O. Box 45327
Omaha, NE 68145
Or, order **TOLL FREE: 800-352-2873**
or online at
www.AddicusBooks.com